Tell Your Dog You're Pregnant

An essential guide for dog owners who are expecting a baby

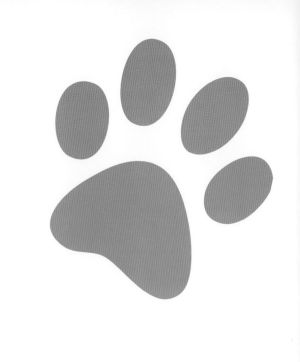

Tell Your Dog You're Pregnant

An essential guide for dog owners who are expecting a baby

By
Dr Lewis Kirkham

BVSc MRCVS CMAVA MANZCVSc(Animal Behaviour)

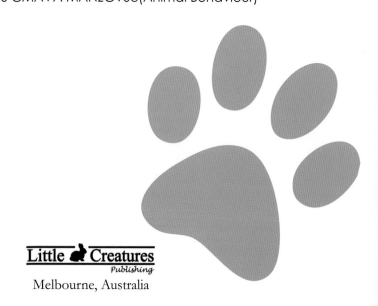

Little Creatures Publishing

Melbourne, Australia

Published by Little Creatures Publishing Pty Ltd (lcp2014pb)
PO Box 777, Port Melbourne, Victoria, Australia 3207
Copyright © Little Creatures Publishing Pty Ltd, 2012

Printed by Everbest Printing / Cover and interior design by Gigi and Lulu / Photos: shutterstock.com

ISBN 978-0-9870530-0-8

National Library of Australia Cataloguing-in-Publication entry:
Kirkham, Lewis.

Tell your dog you're pregnant : an essential guide for dog owners who are expecting a baby /
by Lewis Kirkham.

1st ed.
ISBN 9780987053008 (pbk.)
Dogs--Behavior.
Dogs--Effect of human beings on.
Pregnancy--Popular works.
636.70887

To my wife, Deb,
for her love and care,
her sense of humour
and her ability to always brighten my day

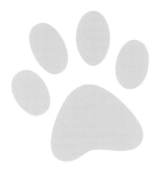

Acknowledgements

My first thanks go to my wife, Deb, who is a constant inspiration and support, and a source of practical advice and profound words of wisdom. Thank you also to my two beautiful daughters, Stella and April, who have shown me how rewarding and fulfilling a (human!) family can be and who generously supplied their baby sounds. I love you both very much. Special thanks go to my parents, Colin and Sonia, for their unconditional love, support, education and editorial input.

This book exists not only because of my stubbornness, but also, and most importantly, because many talented people helped and encouraged me along the way. I would like to thank Dr Robert Holmes and Dr Gabrielle Carter for inspiring and assisting me to pursue my dreams in the field of veterinary behavioural studies and Dr Nick Branson, Dr Debbie Calnon, Dr Caroline Perrin, Dr Diane van Rooy and Professor Paul McGreevy for their professional input.

Thank you also to Nic Redhouse, Leah Horsfall and Nan McNab for their editorial expertise and Graeme Kirkham for his professional advice and his patience with my difficult and repetitive questions. In particular, thank you to Prue Walstab for her vision and project design and Simon Morcom for his printing assistance.

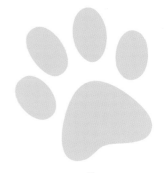

As a paediatrician, parent and dog owner I applaud Dr Kirkham's comprehensive, practical and well-organised approach to introducing a new baby to a resident dog. It is well known to paediatricians that children between the ages of two and five years may have some negative reactions to the homecoming of a new baby, e.g. more demanding behaviour, retrogression in 'toilet training', demanding to be fed by the bottle again, change in sleep patterns and so on. So, just as it makes sense to prepare your existing children for the homecoming of a new baby, so it makes eminent sense to prepare your dog also, because undoubtedly the dog considers itself one of the family, and the consequences, on rare occasions, can be more serious. I thoroughly recommend Dr Kirkham's book to all expectant parents who own a dog. It is perhaps mandatory reading.

Dr Ken Mountain MBBS MPS DCH FRACP
Consultant Paediatrician

Tell Your Dog You're Pregnant contains essential information for expectant parents and carers. It provides clear explanations of how to best prepare your dog while enabling owners to make informed decisions to seek veterinary help early. This could be the key to preventing horrific injuries or possibly saving a baby's life.

Dr Dane Horsfall MBBS(Hons) FACEM
Emergency Physician

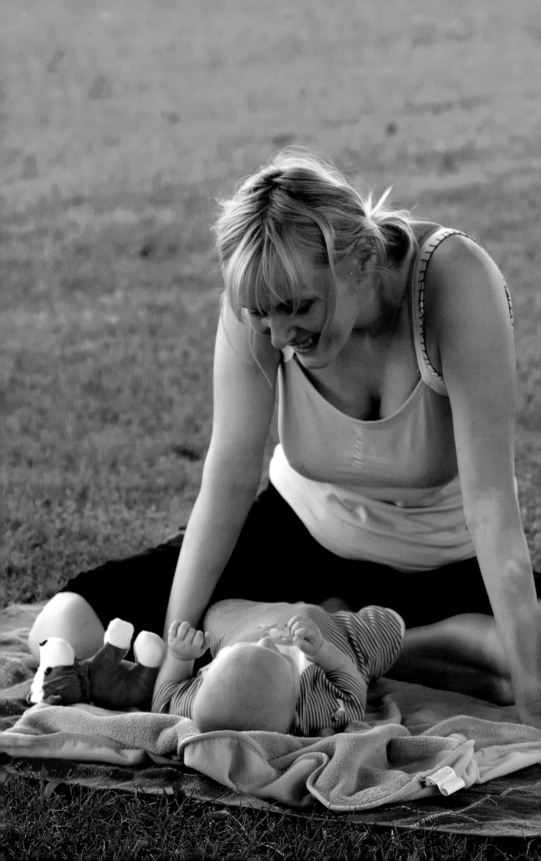

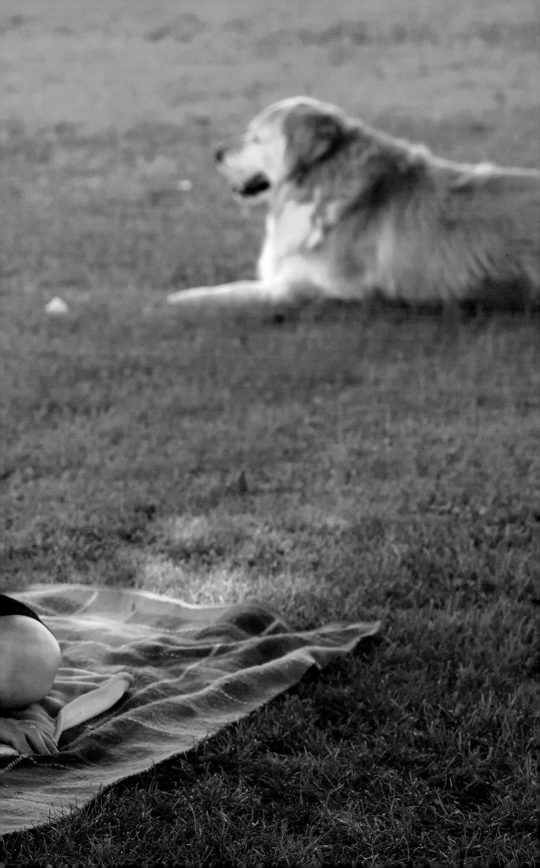

Contents

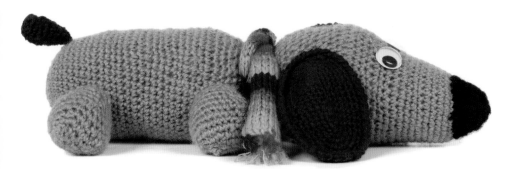

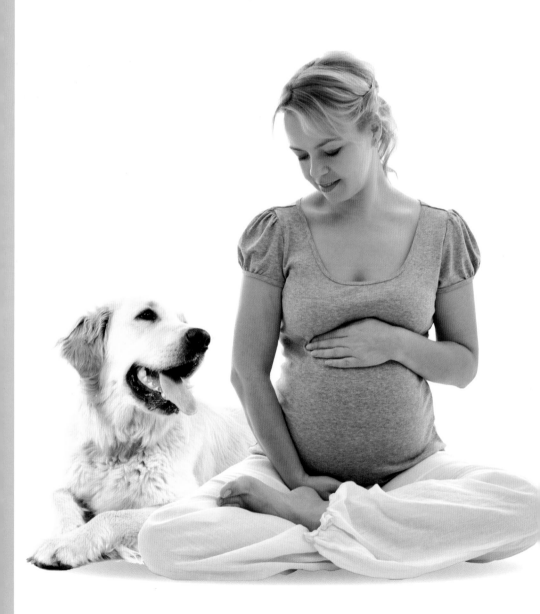

Introduction

Do you have a much-loved dog? Your 'fur kid'? Are you expecting or trying for a baby and want to prepare your pet for this change with minimal stress? This book is designed specifically for you. It comes with a CD containing 13 tracks specifically designed to prepare your dog for your baby's arrival.* Each track contains sounds that will be new to your home when your baby arrives. With the help of the CD and the information in this book, you and your dog will have a more successful and happier transition to a larger family. Remember, dogs that are properly prepared usually adjust to the new addition with few problems.

It is important to read the entire book before playing any of the tracks to your dog. By all means play the sounds to yourself, but not to your dog until you are ready to work through the program.

Early preparation

Whatever stage you are at – whether you are trying for a baby or are due to give birth soon – there are many things you can do in the time remaining to prepare you and your dog for this major change. Preparing early, of course, gives your dog more time to adjust to most of the changes in the household, short of your baby actually arriving. These changes in the household often cause an alteration in a dog's behaviour. If your dog is not adjusting well to these early prenatal household changes, then you will know that it is not the actual presence of your baby that is causing the problems. This book will also help to identify when you may need further professional advice. Any reference in the book to an 'appropriate veterinarian' means veterinarians with a professional interest in animal behaviour.

* The baby and toy sounds can also be downloaded free as MP3 tracks from **http://goo.gl/ZegaeG**

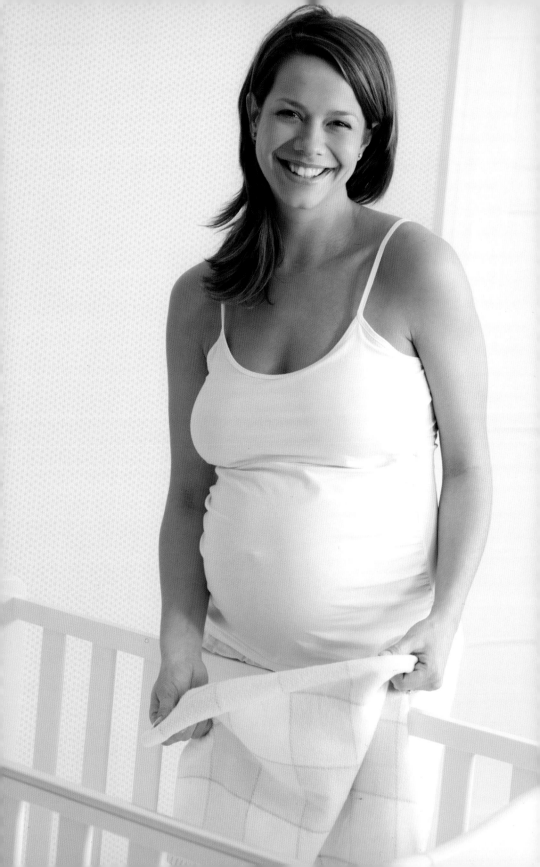

Who needs this book?

If you are an expectant parent as well as a dog owner, this book is for you. From before your baby's birth until roughly their first birthday (when babies become more mobile), you will find helpful advice for managing your dog's interactions with your baby. While many owners find their dog is friendly and gentle around older children or adults, it is very important to keep in mind that dogs can react quite differently to the noises and movements of a small baby.

This book is also helpful if you are likely to have a newborn or small baby as a visitor, whether you are a friend, grandparent, aunt, uncle or other relative of an expectant family; so, remember to pass on the book to any dog owner who is likely to be involved with your new baby. Or, better still, buy them their own copy!

 If prepared in advance, most dogs easily adjust to the arrival of a baby

Your dog and babies

Ask yourself if your dog has had previous exposure to young babies. How did the dog react? If your dog reacted unfavourably, you have some work to do, and you may even require the assistance of a professional. But this book will help. Even if your dog reacts favourably to babies, it is still best to take all relevant precautions, as the consequences of being wrong can be devastating. Do not alarm yourself though; if prepared in advance, most dogs quickly and easily adjust to the arrival of a new baby.

If your dog has never spent much time around babies, it is a good idea to begin exposing them to the sights, sounds and smells of a newborn. While this is a great idea in theory, it is not easy to achieve in practice. This is where *Tell Your Dog You're Pregnant* will greatly assist you.

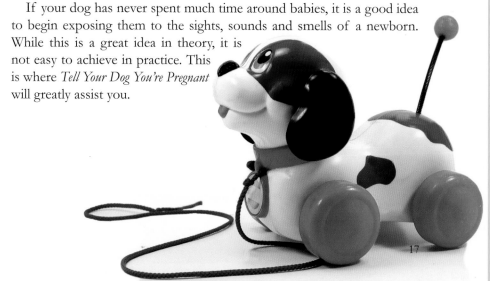

Case study: An active dog with idle paws

A few years ago, I had a phone call from Beth, who was seven months pregnant. She was in a desperate state because she was considering putting her dog to sleep. Rosie, a six-year-old Jack Russell Terrier cross, had always been a handful but her behaviour was becoming progressively worse. Beth did not think she could handle Rosie as well as a new little person in the house. This was causing her terrible distress and guilt. How could she be considering euthanasing Rosie, her much-loved companion?

Unfortunately, Beth is not alone. Every year many pets are surrendered to animal shelters or put to sleep because a baby is being welcomed into the family. Beth clearly did not want Rosie to become one of these statistics.

I arranged a behaviour consultation at Beth's house to assess and discuss Rosie. She was destroying the back garden; she was barking incessantly when her owners were occupied with other activities, such as having friends over or talking on the phone. She did not understand the simplest of commands. I could see why Beth was so upset, however, the situation was not as dire as she thought.

After a long discussion and many questions, the problems with Rosie were very clear. I could see that Rosie was an intelligent dog with an active mind. She was used to being walked each morning before Beth went to work and to enjoying further time in the evenings at the local dog park running, snooping and sniffing her canine friends' bottoms. This all changed when Beth was three months pregnant because she had developed an unstable pelvis and was no longer able to walk Rosie. Although Beth's partner Rob had taken over walking Rosie, he wasn't able to keep up with her usual amounts of exercise due to work commitments.

Beth was dealing with an active dog that had become bored and destructive due to changes in the household even before the baby had arrived. She needed more physical and mental stimulation. What did we do? Rob agreed to walk Rosie four times a week and on the other three days a neighbour who also owned a dog took her to the park.

At home, where Beth could sit down, she started some simple training exercises to engage Rosie's active mind and to help set up predictable interactions between them. I showed them a variety of food release devices/toys to keep Rosie occupied in the backyard as well as other ways of engaging such an active dog. We planned a schedule for all of these activities that could be realistically maintained when their baby arrived. Beth and Rob also used an early version of *Tell Your Dog You're Pregnant* to prepare Rosie for their new family member.

Beth and Rob were dedicated dog owners and Rosie responded well to the training and management. Rosie and the baby, Ben, are great friends. Life is great for Rosie because good things happen whenever Ben is around.

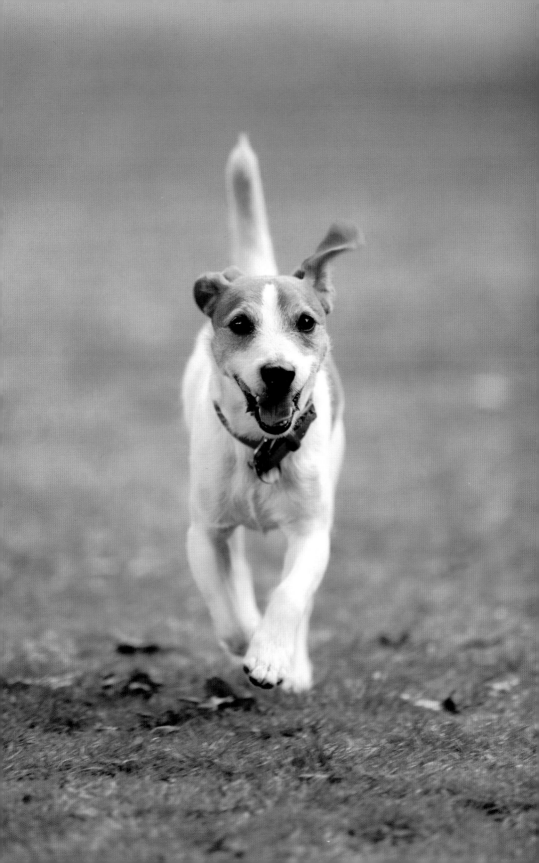

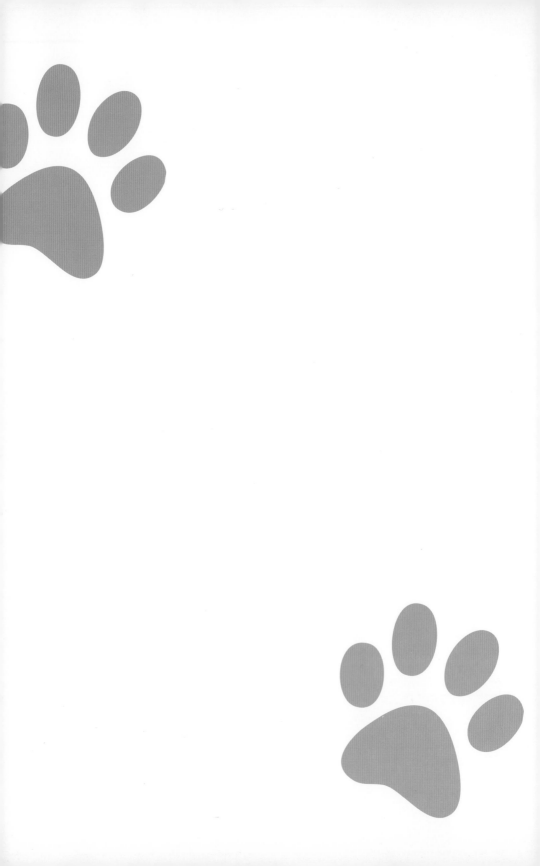

1

Common myths and problems

Common myths exposed

'The dog is jealous ...'

Many dog owners claim the most common emotion displayed by their dog when a baby arrives is jealousy; the dog is 'put out' by the newcomer. In fact, the dog is probably feeling anxious, not jealous. Much of this anxiety is associated with sudden changes to its routine. For this reason, it is important to start preparing your dog as soon as possible for your baby's arrival. The longer lead-time you have to introduce changes to the household, the less disruption there will be when your baby comes home.

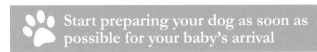

Start preparing your dog as soon as possible for your baby's arrival

'You should spend more time with the dog in preparation for the baby ...'

Many expectant parents feel guilty that they will have less time with their dog when their baby arrives, so they try to increase the number of walks and the amount of attention they give their dog before the baby is born. They hope this will be stored in an 'attention bank' which the dog can draw from once the baby arrives. Unfortunately, this can have the opposite effect; in addition to the new little person disrupting the household, the dog becomes more unsettled as the amount of attention they receive goes from unusually high to minimal overnight.

'The dog will instantly "love" the baby ...'

Aggression from dogs towards newborns is frightening. Not all dogs naturally love babies, or will just 'know that your baby is part of the family'. At the same time, dogs generally do not perceive a baby as a 'threat'. It is the changes within the household that usually cause alterations in a dog's behaviour.

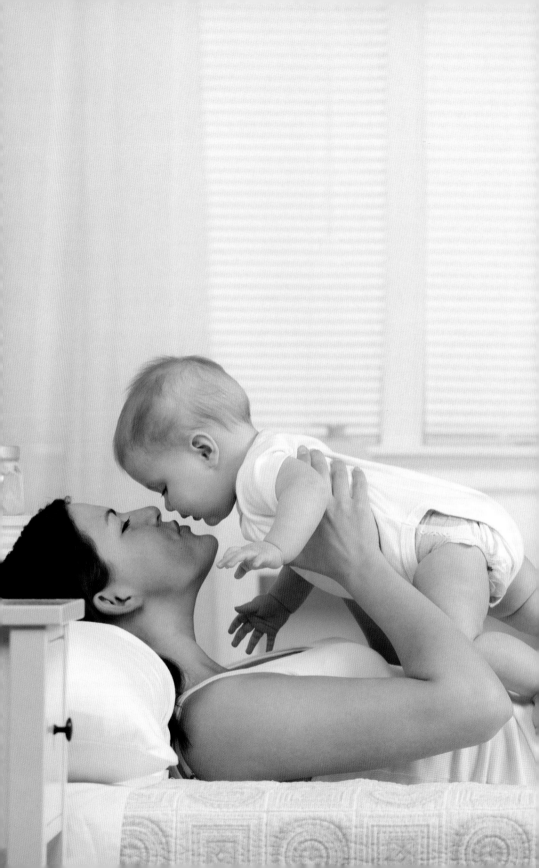

Common problems

'The dog is scared of the baby …'

Some dogs are worried by or even scared of babies. They do not like the sounds, smells and movements babies make, or they are unaccustomed to them. This book specifically details how to prepare your dog for a baby (without a baby actually being present) so the dog is less likely to be fearful when your baby does arrive. It discusses how to create good emotional associations with the baby, rather than fear. It also highlights the early warning signs that may indicate your dog is fearful of your baby, prompting you to seek immediate professional assistance.

'Your dog notices a decrease in attention …'

One of a dog's most enjoyable activities is social contact and attention from its owner. Such contact will decrease once the baby is born. In some cases, this can literally be overnight! This book discusses how to prepare your dog for this change so that the partial loss of a highly valued part of its life is not so dramatic. It will enable your dog to adapt to receiving less attention.

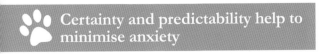

Certainty and predictability help to minimise anxiety

'Interactions have changed and are no longer predictable …'

Once the baby arrives your dog may start to get conflicting signals from you. Your interactions may change and become less predictable. For example, if your dog has always been allowed on your lap it may find that suddenly, when the baby is on your lap, this is no longer allowed. Such a lack of predictability and control over interactions can cause anxiety. This book will help you set up predictable interactions before the baby arrives and enable you to make changes early on that give your dog a clear understanding of what it should be doing in certain situations. Certainty and predictability help to minimise any anxiety.

Case study: You're in my seat!

I went to visit Kate, who had a three-week-old baby, Annabelle. Her dog Rastus, a nine-year-old Poodle, had developed some unpleasant habits since Annabelle had arrived on the scene.

Of course, all new mums want feeding times with a newborn to be peaceful and uninterrupted. Unfortunately, whenever Kate sat on the couch to feed Annabelle, Rastus would disturb them by trying to jump up on Kate's lap. Annabelle would become distressed and wouldn't feed.

Kate became frustrated with what appeared to be Rastus's jealousy and banished Rastus to the backyard where he barked, howled and whined, just to make sure the neighbours knew how horribly he was being treated. If Kate wasn't able to put him outside, she would lock him in the laundry where he would scratch at the door and become destructive.

After chatting with Kate and observing Rastus, it was apparent to me that he was quite anxious about the activities in the house. Prior to Annabelle's arrival, Kate had been on maternity leave for five weeks. During this time, she and Rastus had spent most afternoons on the couch, reading or enjoying a long nap. Rastus was clearly missing the special afternoon time he had with Kate. He had no idea what he should be doing now that Annabelle had arrived. Contrary to popular belief, Rastus was not barking and howling and being destructive to spite her, rather he was anxious at being separated from Kate – he just couldn't help it.

We got Rastus his own special mat to sit on during Annabelle's feeding times. Kate would give him a bone or chewy treat on the mat to keep him occupied. He could then be close to Kate but also enjoy a tasty food reward at the same time. Kate would occasionally throw a tasty treat towards Rastus to encourage his new quiet behaviour.

Rastus now looks forward to these baby feeding times. In the evening, when Kate's partner is home, we ensured she schedule some 'Rastus time' where he was allowed onto her lap for his own dedicated time of grooming and cuddles.

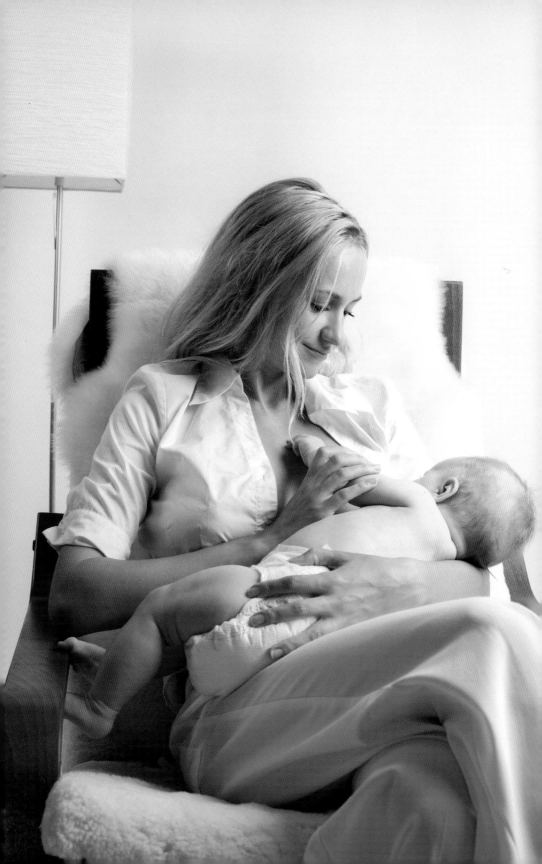

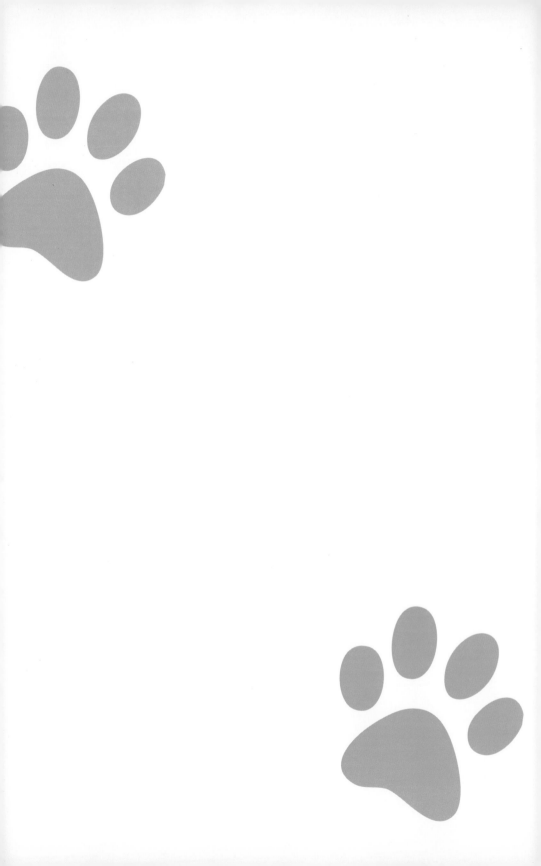

2

Training, supervising and separating

Training

Once you have a baby, it is even more important that you are able to control your dog, especially when you are at a distance from them or have your arms full. The old saying, 'You can't teach an old dog new tricks' is a myth. It is more likely that your dog has a lot of ingrained 'old tricks' that need to be trained out before they can learn these 'new tricks'.

 The recommended commands: sit, stay, come, drop it and go to your mat

Responding to commands

Your dog needs to respond reliably to at least five simple instructions: sit, stay, come, drop it, and go to your mat or bed. There are others, but these are the minimum requirements. If these five commands are not in your dog's repertoire, or your dog only responds intermittently, or you need to raise your voice to get a response, you should seek the assistance of a professional dog trainer. Ideally, you want your dog to respond correctly after one request, without the need to raise your voice. Yelling the same word repeatedly, increasingly loudly, does not usually increase the chance of your dog responding favourably. (This is the same for children, too!) Your dog may be 'grand champion' at the local obedience club, but you need to ensure that they will respond to you at home. If you have more than one dog, then each dog should respond when alone and when together.

 Reward your dog when they are calm and quiet

Rewarding good behaviour

Start rewarding your dog when they are calm and quiet. This may mean whispering quietly 'good dog' to them while resting, or surprising them with a chew toy while they are lounging in the sun. Encouraging calm, quiet behaviour is very important as you will need periods like this once your baby arrives.

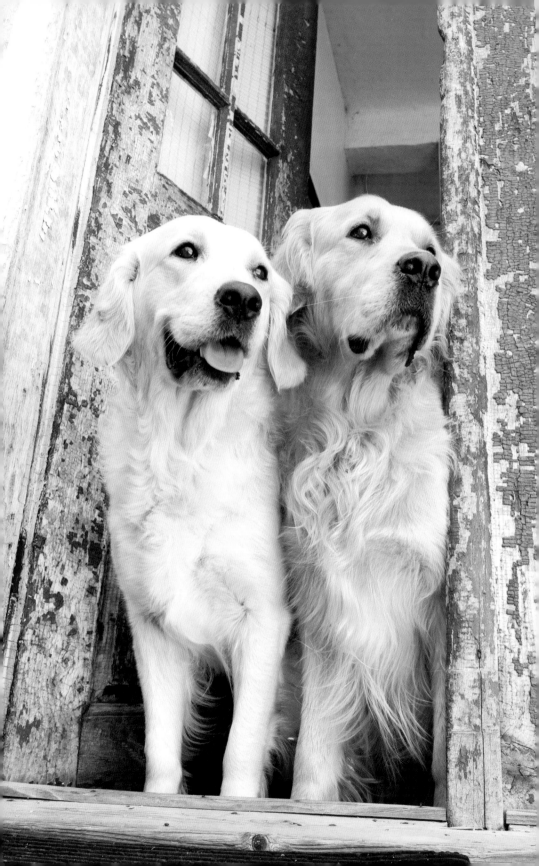

Training methods

Currently, you may be using physical or verbal corrections or punishment to reprimand or obtain obedience from your dog. These methods are not suitable within a family. Babies and children are physically and mentally unable to interact successfully with a dog by using physical or verbal commands or corrections. Furthermore, these methods do not create a harmonious home environment in which a child-dog relationship can develop.

The training methods you use should be effective for the entire family and should be based on rewarding desirable behaviours and ignoring or redirecting unfavourable behaviours. To make sure the relationship between your dog and baby is a happy one, good things need to occur whenever your baby is around.

 The training methods you use should be effective for the entire family

Toilet training

If your dog is not well toilet trained, now is a good time to recommence training. You may also need to retrain your dog to toilet in a different area if the current location is inconvenient. Slipping on a mess in the middle of the night as you rush to tend to your baby is not fun! You also do not want messes in a place where your baby may roll or crawl.

See **www.babyandpet.com.au** for specific help with toilet training.

Owning two or more dogs

If you have two or more dogs in the house, you will know that each has a different personality. It is advisable to perform all the assessments and training outlined in this book with each dog separately to ascertain their individual reaction before reassessing all the dogs together. This includes steps 1 to 5 described later (with the sounds) and the initial introductions when your baby first arrives home.

Consider also how your dogs currently interact with each other, and how this could affect a new baby. Some dogs chase each other, playing loudly and roughly. Other dogs fight over certain items or areas within a household. This can include food, bones, toys, attention and resting places. Any fights between dogs could be a problem if your baby gets caught in between. These issues need to be addressed early on, and if necessary discussed with an appropriate veterinarian.

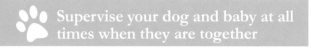
Supervise your dog and baby at all times when they are together

Supervision

This book and its associated training methods and techniques do not replace the need for constant adult supervision of your baby and dog. What is constant adult supervision? It means that if your dog and baby are in the same room, or near each other, then you should be present, attentive and at all times no more than an arm's length from your baby or your dog, or both. This applies even when one or both of them are asleep.

If you cannot supervise their interactions closely enough, you need to separate your dog and your child until you are again able to monitor them closely. If your dog currently exhibits aggression towards babies, or you are unsure how to interpret your dog's behaviour, seek assistance from an appropriate veterinarian.

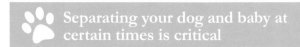
Separating your dog and baby at certain times is critical

Separation

Mention is made throughout this book of the need to place your dog in a 'safe and secure area' or 'separate your dog from your baby'. **Separation is different from supervision.** Separation means that there is a physical barrier between your dog and the baby that cannot be breached by either of them. This usually means a closed solid door, preferably with a lock. The lock should prevent anyone inadvertently opening the door, such as older children or unsuspecting visitors. This means that your dog and baby are separated until you are available to adequately supervise them again. The physical barrier should not allow a child to place a hand through the barrier into the dog's space. Barriers, baby gates or playpens that can be leapt over by the dog, and doors that do not properly close, are not suitable for separation.

The benefits of your best friend

Social benefits

The family benefits of owning a pet are numerous and well documented.
- Studies have shown that children who own dogs are less self-centred, have higher self-esteem, have greater empathy and are more caring.

- Dogs are often seen as stable friends to children; they offer unconditional love during difficult times.
- Research shows that children who own dogs are more popular with their peers, have better communication and social skills and develop friendships more easily. Owning a dog decreases feelings of loneliness.
- Caring for a dog creates a sense of responsibility and encourages a daily care and exercise routine.
- Owning a dog can also assist in teaching about life and death.
- As well as providing a constant source of enjoyment, friendship, companionship and fun, many dogs thrive in a family environment.

Health benefits

- Children who own dogs are more active and less likely to be overweight.
- Studies have shown that dog owners suffer fewer headaches, colds and hay fever, and visit the doctor less often.
- Research shows that adults who own a dog have lower stress levels, lower heart rates and lower blood pressure – all common ailments for a new parent!
- You have a better chance of surviving a heart attack if you own a dog.
- Owning a dog has also been shown to assist in lowering cholesterol levels.

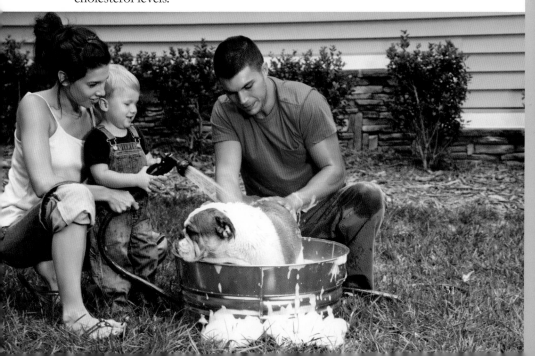

Case study: There's a stork at the front door!

Barney was a seven-year-old Labrador. He was a lovely dog but he went crazy whenever the doorbell rang. He would charge to the front door and bark loudly. His owners, Tania and James, had been tolerant of Barney's noisy behaviour but now they were expecting a baby in a few months, and they were worried.

The nursery was right next to the front door. Tania could imagine her peacefully sleeping baby being startled and upset by Barney's behaviour. There was also the risk that Barney could hurt someone if they were in the hallway carrying the baby when the doorbell rang.

A new baby attracts many visitors and deliveries – the doorbell would be chiming every day, possibly several times a day. Tania rang me to arrange a house call.

True to form, when I rang the doorbell, Barney greeted me hysterically from behind the front door. His bark was loud – I was sure it would wake a baby in the next street let alone in the next room!

James, who was obviously used to the noise, opened the front door, smiled knowingly and gestured for me to enter. He knew not to try to speak as words would have been futile with such a racket. The way Barney answered the door was definitely a problem.

I discussed with Tania and James that we needed to change Barney's association with the doorbell. Currently, he knew that when it rang it meant visitors and often excitement and attention for him. In this way, every time he greeted someone at the door he was rewarded. This training would take some time, but thankfully Tania's baby was not due for a while.

Tania and James started working on some basic obedience for Barney using food rewards. This gave them better control over his behaviour at times when the doorbell was not ringing. Then we needed to change his response to the doorbell by training him to seek out his owners when the doorbell rang rather than charging up the hallway. Fortunately, being a Labrador, Barney was motivated by food rewards. Several elevated containers of treats were placed strategically around the house, so that when the doorbell rang, Tania or James could call him over for a treat, which enabled them to have better control over him during these times.

Barney needed lots of practice and lots of doorbell rings from pretend visitors. Fortunately, one of Tania's neighbours, Marilyn, was also motivated by food rewards (Belgian chocolate and champagne to be exact). When bribed with these treats, Marilyn was more than happy to ring the doorbell, enabling dedicated training times. After a while, she then agreed to visit at random times to mimic more realistic visitor arrivals.

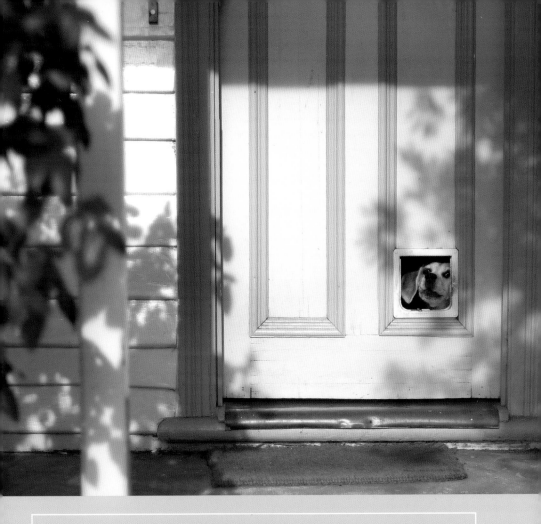

Consistency and repetition were the key to Barney's success: Tania and James needed to follow the same routine every time the doorbell rang to alter Barney's greeting behaviour.

Eight months later baby Jacob was born and I made a surprise visit to check on Barney's progress. I walked up to the front porch and rang the doorbell with some trepidation. Nothing happened – there was silence. I waited for a minute or so and when there was no noise at the door, I walked out the gate, assuming nobody was home. Just as I was leaving, the front door opened and Tania waved and beckoned for me to come in. She whispered that she had just settled Jacob to sleep. My concern was for Barney – he was nowhere in sight. As I entered the living room my eyes lit up – James was sitting on the couch watching TV (with the volume turned up very loud) while Barney was looking up at him expectantly for a tasty food reward. Barney had heard the doorbell but clearly James had not!

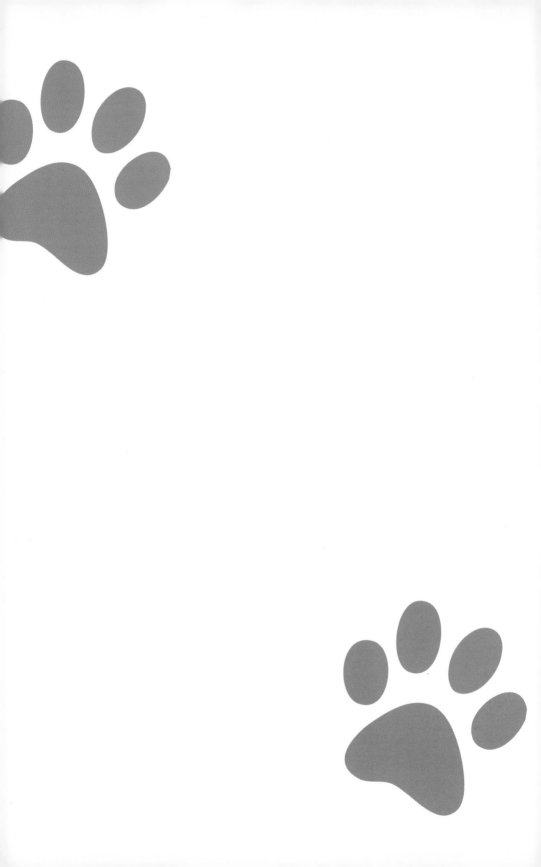

3
Dog bites

The hard facts

While owning a dog can be a delightful family experience with enormous benefits for the child and the parents; families and carers need to be aware of the risk of injury from dog bites.

- A common misconception is that most dog bites occur on the street from 'stray dogs'. This is far from the case. Approximately 70 per cent of all bites occur in or around the home and are from a dog familiar to the child. This may be a dog belonging to you, a friend or a neighbour. More than half of all dog bites are related to innocuous activities such as playing with or near a dog, cuddling or feeding a dog and walking past a dog.
- Children are usually bitten on the head, face or neck, and can be left with permanent scarring – both physical and emotional. Post-traumatic stress disorder is seen in 55 per cent of children after a substantial bite.
- Generally, a bite from a larger dog will cause greater damage, and such bites make up the majority of dog-related emergency hospital admissions.

 Any breed of dog can bite

- Any breed of dog can bite, and every individual dog can bite, even those that appear exceptionally friendly or 'have never bitten'. In one study, two-thirds of reported dog-bite incidents were from dogs that had 'never previously bitten a child'.
- A child is twice as likely as an adult to be bitten by a dog.
- Almost half of all children will have been bitten by a dog by the time they are 18, and approximately one-fifth of these will require medical attention. Many adults can remember being bitten by a dog as a child.
- Children under five years of age are the most likely to be bitten and smaller children are often more seriously injured. Horrifically, fatalities from dog attacks do occur, ranging from one to two fatalities per year in Australia to 30 fatalities per year in the United States.

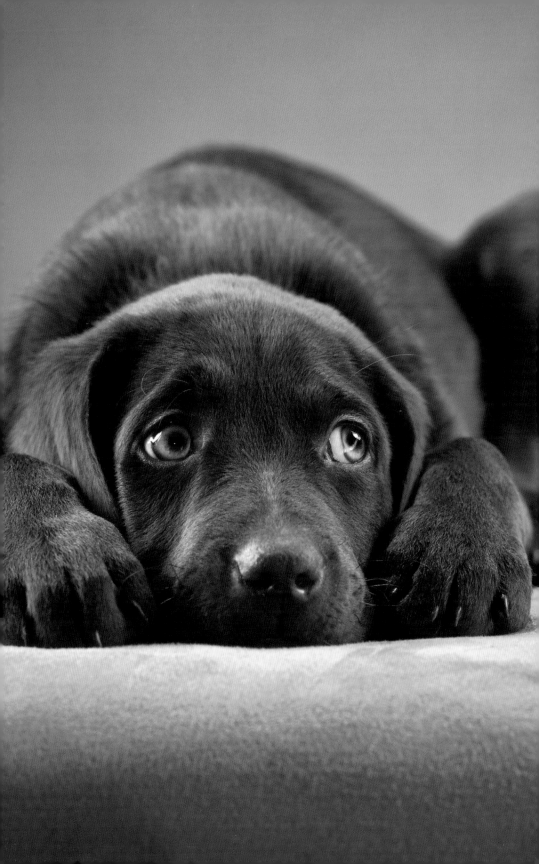

Why might a dog bite?

Dogs can bite for a variety of reasons. Summarised below are the common reasons why a dog may become aggressive when a baby arrives. But do not be alarmed; one of the main objectives of this book is to reduce the chance of problems occurring. This book will help you identify early warning signs that your dog and new baby may not get along, enabling you to seek professional assistance.

 An aim of this book is to reduce the chance of problems occuring

Fear

Aggression directed towards newborns is not usually associated with jealousy, or being 'put out', or an urge to dominate. Depending on early experiences, previous contact with babies or individual temperaments, some dogs can actually be afraid of babies and the noises or movements they make. This fear can be seen as (permanent) avoidance or sometimes aggression.

Loss of attention

A sudden loss of highly valued attention from the owner (or social contact) can cause a dog to be aggressive. This can occur when a baby arrives home. If a dog perceives that there is a threat to this valued attention, they may try to regain some of these desirable interactions by being aggressive.

Conflict

Conflict can occur within a dog's mind when they are unsure of what behaviour they should be showing in certain situations. This is different from the human emotion 'jealousy'. It can be caused by a lack of predictability and control over what happens within a dog's environment. This can result from the large number of changes that occur within a house once a baby arrives. Often a dog becomes unsure about what is the correct thing to do to get a reward (attention, treats) from the owner and this creates conflict for the dog. For example, conflict could occur if your dog usually sits on your lap whenever you are on the couch, but now that you are nursing a baby, your dog is told off for trying to get onto your lap.

Resource guarding

Some dogs may become aggressive if they are approached when they have a bone or toy or some other item they adore. Other dogs can become protective of an area (for example, their owner's bed) and become aggressive when approached or touched while in that area.

Tethering or tying up

Tying your dog up outside (or inside) for long periods is also a risk factor for children being bitten. Dogs can be protective of their restricted space when tied up and become aggressive when children stray into their area. For this reason tying your dog to a post or tree or tethering them to a long line for extended periods is not recommended. If you feel you must tie up your dog, consider the reasons behind the need for doing so before your baby arrives and find an alternative solution.

Instinct

A very small number of dogs may display predatory aggression towards a baby. These dogs may or may not have hunted, caught and killed small animals or birds in the past. Although there is no definitive link, there is some thought that certain dogs could mistake a crying, wriggling baby for prey. This does not mean that if your dog has caught birds or small animals in the past they will definitely be aggressive to your baby, but rather that you need to be more vigilant of your dog's responses to your baby. If your dog exhibits predatory behaviour towards babies (for example, stalking, strong focus, strange whining or unusual interest), or you are concerned that this might be the case, seek assistance from an appropriate veterinarian.

Separation anxiety and noise phobias

Recent scientific research indicates that approximately three-quarters of dogs with a history of biting children, when presented to a particular veterinary behaviour clinic, also showed signs of separation anxiety or noise-related phobias or both. This research indicates that if your dog has problems with separation anxiety or has a phobia about noises or thunderstorms, then your dog may be at greater risk of biting your child. You should consider treating your dog for these conditions before your baby arrives.

Signs of separation anxiety vary. Such signs usually only occur when the dog is separated from their owners. This may be when the owner is not home and the dog is alone or simply when the dog is separated from the owner by a door. It can even occur when the dog can see the owner through the door!

Signs of noise-related phobias are similar to those for separation anxiety but only occur when the dog hears a particular noise. Common noises that cause anxiety are thunderstorms, fireworks, vacuum cleaners, loud trucks and construction sites.

Common signs of both these conditions are shaking, drooling, hiding, panting, pacing, barking or howling, scratching and chewing at doors or windows, escaping, destruction and house-soiling. If you are unsure whether your dog suffers from these conditions or you require assistance in treating these problems, seek advice from an appropriate veterinarian.

Pain or illness

An illness or painful condition can make a dog act aggressively. Common ailments are skin and ear problems, arthritis and dental issues. Any illness in your dog should be promptly addressed by your veterinarian.

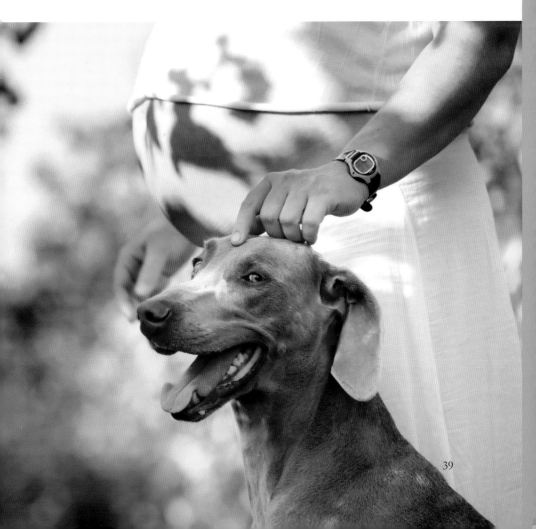

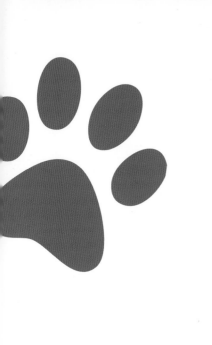

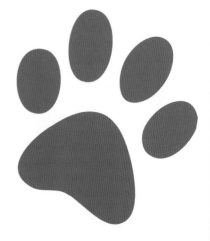

4

Preparing your dog

A well-prepared dog is more likely to accept a new baby without problems. The first step is to know your dog and how it is likely to react to something new and strange. The next step is to prepare your dog carefully, and well in advance, for the arrival of your new baby.

How to assess your dog's behaviour

There are many subtle variations in canine body language. Outlined below are some signs to watch for that will assist you in assessing your dog's demeanour. Some are obvious, others are subtle. These signs are listed below in **behaviour groups A, B and C**, which aim to give you a general appreciation of your dog's current emotional state. While playing the CD sounds, observe your dog and identify their reaction using the behaviour groups. The behaviour groups can also be used to assess your dog's possible emotional state in other situations.

Assessment based purely on these three behaviour groups is not a substitute for seeking professional advice. If you are having trouble assessing your dog's behavioural signs then seek the help of an appropriate veterinarian.

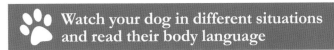

Watch your dog in different situations and read their body language

Reading your dog's body language

You need to be able to read your dog's body language. Watch your dog closely in many different situations and see what they do. For example, do they put their ears down when they meet another dog, wag their tail or raise their hackles and stand tall? At all times when assessing your dog, try to put yourself in their shoes (or paws) and determine if your dog is comfortable and relaxed. Trust your instincts; you know your dog, and if something does not feel right about your dog's behaviour, either towards the CD sounds or towards your baby, then it probably isn't right. It is better to seek professional advice from an appropriate veterinarian and be sure, rather than be sorry later.

Never punish or reprimand your dog for displaying any behavioural signs even if you consider them to be inappropriate – this is how they communicate their feelings. Some of these signs are helpful warnings that your dog may not be completely relaxed and that you need to remove your dog from the situation. If the signs persist, you need to seek assistance from an appropriate veterinarian.

Behaviour groups

Use the signs listed in these behaviour groups to assess your dog. Every dog has individual behavioural responses and body language. The signs should only be used as a guide to your dog's current emotional state. But you can use the behaviour group signs to assess your dog in any situation – not just when playing the tracks.

Behaviour group A

Your dog may exhibit *one or more* of these signs, indicating that they may be alert or mildly inquisitive in the current situation (for example, when a track is played or your baby is present). These signs are generally non-threatening and not usually a concern, but your dog should be monitored to ensure they do not develop into signs outlined in behaviour groups B or C.
- Ears pointing up and forwards (pricking of ears)
- Head cocked to the side, as if listening
- Sniffing (particularly the ground)
- Looking at the speakers or the source of the sound
- Moving slowly towards the object or sound

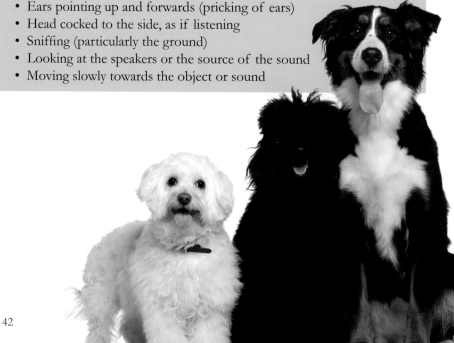

Behaviour group B

Your dog may exhibit *one or more* of these signs, indicating that they may be uncomfortable or anxious in the current situation.

- Yawning
- Licking their lips or nose
- Furrowed or worried brow line
- Slow blinking
- Dilated pupils
- Eyes darting from side to side
- Looking sideways so you can see the whites of their eyes
- Appearing to fall asleep (or drowsiness) while sitting or standing
- Ears pointing sideways (or at right angles to their head)
- Looking away and turning their head away
- Lowered head and body, or cowering
- Backing away
- Very still and tense body
- Suddenly scratching, licking, biting or grooming themselves
- Shaking or shivering as if cold
- Excessive panting or even panting when not obviously hot
- Tail low or tucked between their legs and still
- Whining or whimpering

Behaviour group C

Your dog may exhibit *one or more* of these signs, indicating that they may be very anxious or fearful in the current situation and may become aggressive. These are serious signs, and your dog should be removed from the situation immediately.

- Staring
- Baring teeth
- Raising or curling their lip
- Ears flat, pointing backwards against their head
- Raised fur on their back and neck (hackles)
- Standing at full height and leaning forward with a tense posture
- Barking
- Snarling, growling or low-pitched grumbling
- Snapping or biting
- Lunging or pulling (on the lead) with or without barking
- Hiding and being non-responsive
- Non-responsive to your requests or to food
- Tail raised high over their back, wagging stiffly

Why play baby sounds to my dog?

A dog's hearing is much more sensitive than a human's, especially to higher-pitched sounds such as a baby crying. Unfamiliar sounds and noises can easily cause excitement, anxiety, agitation, nervousness, and fear in any dog. They can also make your dog howl or bark. This is especially true if your dog is already reactive to certain noises (for example, thunderstorms or fireworks). These types of responses are common and can make for a difficult introduction to your baby. There are some dogs that howl like a wolf when they first hear a baby's cry! Clearly this sort of response has the potential to upset you and your new baby.

Playing these tracks now, before the baby arrives, will indicate whether your dog is likely to react unfavourably to baby noises. By playing the tracks and following a series of steps (steps 1 to 5) outlined later in this chapter, your dog will become accustomed to the sounds associated with a new baby and this will help in reducing any unfavourable responses.

 Observe closely how your dog reacts to the sounds

Playing the tracks*

So as not to worsen your dog's responses to these new noises, it is important to introduce the sounds gradually, as described later in steps 1 to 5. Likewise, it is very important to observe closely how your dog is reacting to the sounds. Pay attention to your dog's behaviour and body language while the sounds are playing. By observing your dog's body language you will be able to work out which one of three behaviour groups (A, B or C) it fits into.

After completing steps 1 to 5 and monitoring your dog's response using the behaviour groups, your dog will be well prepared for the different sounds and noises that accompany a new baby. You will also be able to identify potential problems and know if you need assistance from an appropriate veterinarian.

Remember, if you have two or more dogs, perform all assessments and training outlined in this book with each dog separately to ascertain their individual reaction before repeating the assessment with all dogs together. This includes steps 1 to 5 (with the sounds) and the initial introductions when your baby arrives home.

* The baby and toy sounds can also be downloaded free as MP3 tracks from **http://goo.gl/ZegaeG**

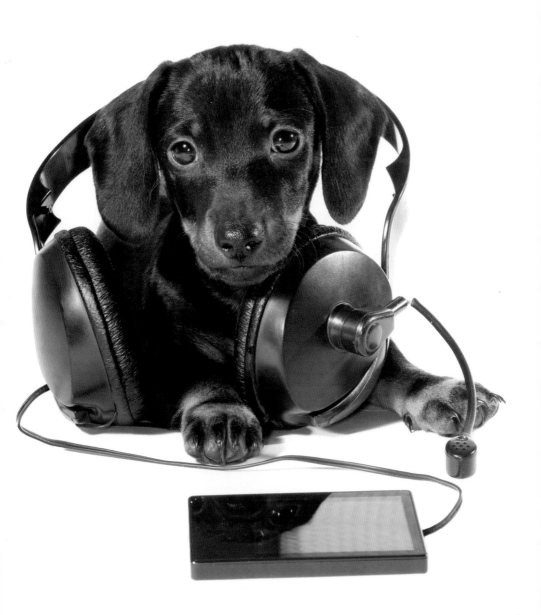

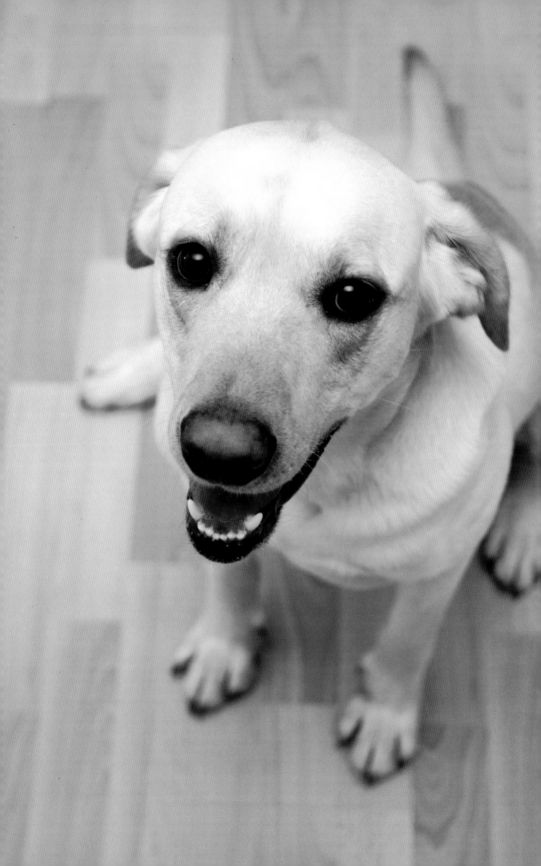

Using the sounds and observing

Before playing any of the tracks to your dog, it is important to read the entire book. By all means play the sounds to yourself, but **not** to your dog until you are ready to follow steps 1 to 5 outlined below.

- Do not attempt to complete all of the steps in one day or even just a week. Take your time over a period of weeks and advance to the next step only when your dog is relaxed and calm.
- Start with several short training sessions (for example, five to ten minutes) and lengthen them gradually; your dog needs time to adjust to the new sounds.
- Your dog's response may depend on the quality of your speakers, so try to use the best quality stereo system available.
- For step 1 (the observation step), play all 13 tracks consecutively at a real-life volume. This enables you to judge your dog's current response to baby and toy sounds.
- Steps 2 to 5 explain how to best prepare your dog for the sounds and routines associated with a baby.
- For steps 2 and 3 the tracks are initially played at a very low volume that does not cause a fearful response in your dog. The volume is slowly and gradually increased over a period of weeks. Play the tracks while you are doing something very enjoyable and highly distracting with your dog. Essentially, you want the sounds to be associated with good things rather than something scary. During these steps it is very important to monitor the behaviour group signs to ensure your dog is comfortable and relaxed at all times.

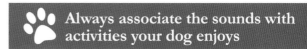
Always associate the sounds with activities your dog enjoys

- In steps 4 and 5 you are setting up household routines that will occur when your baby arrives. These routines create certainty and predictability in both your mind and your dog's mind, which help to lower (everyone's!) anxiety.
- Steps 4 and 5 will also highlight certain situations that may require further assistance from an appropriate veterinarian.

The 5 steps

 Step 1: Play all the sounds at a real-life volume once only. Observe and assess your dog

Step 1

This is an observation step. **Only perform this step once.** Performing this step more than once can worsen a dog's response to the sounds.

Play all the tracks at a *real-life* volume. While the tracks are playing, observe your dog and gauge their reaction. Do not try to excite your dog or even direct them towards the sounds. Just play the tracks and observe.

Some dogs will not respond to the tracks. They will show none of the signs outlined in behaviour groups A, B or C and will act as if they have not even heard the sounds. Assuming that your dog's hearing is normal, then this lack of response can be attributed to one of two reasons:

- either your dog is not bothered by the sounds of babies; or
- your dog does not associate the sounds coming from a stereo system with real baby sounds. In this case your dog may only respond to the noises of a baby when a real baby is present.

If your dog does not respond to the sounds, go to step 4. You will need to monitor your dog's behavioural responses more closely when they hear your actual baby for the first time. If they respond unfavourably (behaviour groups B or C) to your actual baby's noises, you will need to seek the assistance of an appropriate veterinarian.

If your dog shows any of the behaviour signs outlined in behaviour groups A, B or C while playing the tracks, move to step 2. Even if your dog responds to just one track or to several of the tracks, move to step 2.

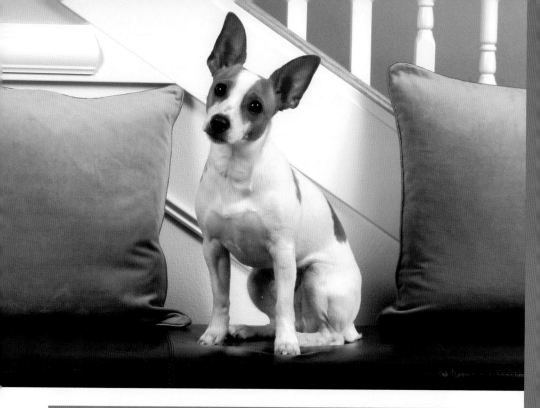

 Step 2: Do something your dog enjoys while playing the sounds at a very low volume

Step 2

Your dog is reacting to the sounds. This is common. Now, replay, at the *lowest audible volume*, each individual track that caused your dog to react. Remember, your dog's hearing is extremely sensitive. While each track is playing, do something really fun with your dog. You will know what your dog enjoys. For many dogs, it is meal time or food rewards; for other dogs, it is playing with their favourite tug toy, or grooming or patting. You want your dog to associate good things with the sounds, and every time a baby sound is heard you want it to be a positive experience. You should be able to distract your dog, so they no longer display the signs outlined in behaviour groups A, B or C while the tracks are playing. Play the tracks several times a day, at the lowest volume, while doing an enjoyable activity.

Continue doing this until your dog appears to be ignoring the sounds or prefers to focus on you and shows none of the signs in behaviour groups A, B or C. Now go to step 3.

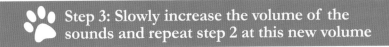

Step 3: Slowly increase the volume of the sounds and repeat step 2 at this new volume

Step 3

Congratulations! Your dog no longer reacts to any of the tracks being played at the *lowest audible volume*. Next, *slowly* increase the volume of each individual track. For each slight increase in volume, do something fun with your dog while the track is playing (as outlined in step 2). Repeat this until your dog appears to be ignoring the sounds or prefers to focus on you and shows none of the signs in behaviour groups A, B or C. Continue to increase the volume gradually, until it is at a volume that you would expect in a real-life situation. Obviously the feeding and bath time tracks need to be quieter.

Remember, babies can scream at around 110dB, which is similar to an ambulance siren or a motorcycle! Babies' cries have a high pitch, so ensure the treble is turned to high on your sound system, not the bass.

Play the tracks at different times of the day and night. Babies' cries *always* sound louder to tired parents in the middle of the night!

When your dog no longer displays the signs outlined in behaviour groups A, B or C, or can easily be distracted by you when any of the tracks are played at real-life volume levels, go to step 4.

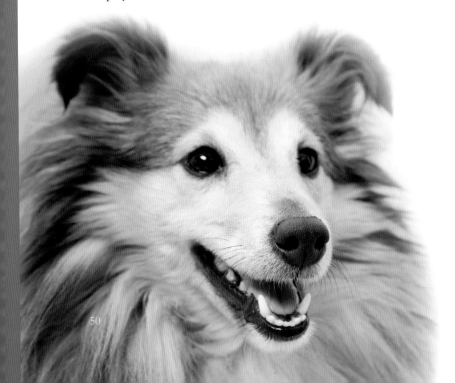

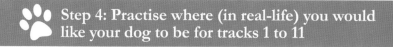
Step 4: Practise where (in real-life) you would like your dog to be for tracks 1 to 11

Step 4

Up until now you should have been playing all 13 tracks on the CD. Step 4 involves using only tracks 1 to 11. Each of these tracks is a sound from a specific situation that will occur with your baby every day. For each track, set up the scenario of where you will be, where your baby will be and what your dog will be doing. For instance, baby feeding time may be on the couch with your baby on your lap. Where will your dog be? Obviously, they cannot be on your lap too. Decide now where you would like your dog to be, and start training them to go to that area at this time. It may be as simple as providing a mat for your dog next to the couch and giving a long-lasting tasty treat in this area to encourage them to remain there while you feed. You may need to do this in several rooms, just as some activities will occur in different rooms. Also, play the tracks in a separate room from where you and your dog are, as your baby will not always be in the same room as you.

New parents often move suddenly and appear anxious when their baby starts crying. When you play the track of a baby crying or screaming in another room, it can be useful to get up suddenly and rush towards the sound. At the same time throw your dog a tasty food treat. These sudden movements and associated food rewards will prepare your dog for your likely movements when your baby starts crying.

If you are going to use a baby monitor, play the tracks through this as well, to accustom your dog to the noise coming from different areas in the house as well as the different quality of sound.

Step 4 may require a longer period of time and more effort, depending on your dog's temperament and 'trainability'. This step sets up a clear routine for you and your dog for what you both should be doing at certain times. This consistency helps lower unpredictability and stress in the dog's environment. Once you have each scenario worked out for tracks 1 to 11, continue to step 5.

Step 5

Add a pretend baby to what you did in step 4. This may be a doll or a teddy bear, or even just a large rolled-up towel or a cushion wrapped in a blanket. This may feel like a strange thing to do, but it enables you to practise the same scenarios as in step 4, but now with your hands full.

Currently, all baby talk in the house is probably directed at your dog (or your partner …). This is going to change! Start talking baby talk to the pretend baby, and more adult-style talk to your dog. This will get your dog used to baby language being used for others in the house as well.

When you finish this step, you should be able to play the first 11 tracks at real-life volume, have a 'baby' in your arms, coo and talk sweet nothings to your 'baby' while your dog is behaving as requested. Your dog is now ready for the sounds of your real baby.

If you get stuck at step 2 or 3, or your dog is consistently displaying concerning behaviours (behaviour group B or C), you need the assistance of an appropriate veterinarian.

There may be other everyday sounds that cause your dog to react unfavourably. These might be the doorbell, telephone, car keys, or the TV. You probably won't want your dog barking madly when it hears the doorbell or telephone when you have just put your baby down for a nap! Record these sounds and proceed through steps 2 and 3 to decrease your dog's response to the noise. You may want to retrain your dog to respond differently to the sound; for instance, going to their mat for a treat when the doorbell rings.

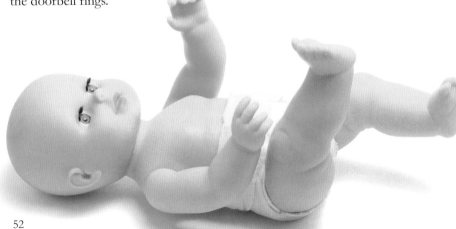

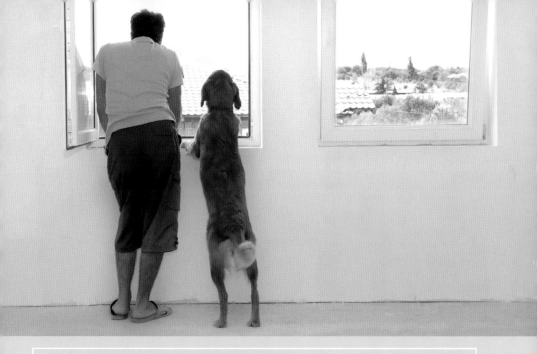

Case study: Who needs training?

John and Penny called me when Penny was three months pregnant. They were concerned about how Molly, their eight-year-old Golden Retriever, was going to react to the new addition. I met them all at their house where we discussed many things, including how to manage several issues that were concerning John and Penny.

Halfway through the consultation, I started to discuss the use of baby and toy sounds to help with Molly's preparation. I took them through the steps and behaviour groups as outlined in *Tell Your Dog You're Pregnant*. After this I suggested we trial the sounds from the CD to see how Molly would react. John inserted the CD into the stereo system and the sounds began to play.

I focused on Molly to monitor her behaviour and assess her response to the sounds, but this focus quickly switched to John, who proceeded to jump and prance around in front of Molly, saying in a high-pitched excited voice, 'What's that Molly? What's that noise, eh, Molly?' and best of all, 'Where's the baby Molly? Get the baby, Molly!'

After calming John down by asking him to stop the CD, I then explained to him that we really did not want Molly to get excited and start searching for the baby whenever she heard a cry. To his credit, John was slightly embarrassed. It was then that my focus switched back to Molly, who had thankfully ignored John's antics and walked into the kitchen to get a drink. I could tell that, with a little bit of work, Molly was going to adapt just fine, but I wasn't so sure about John!

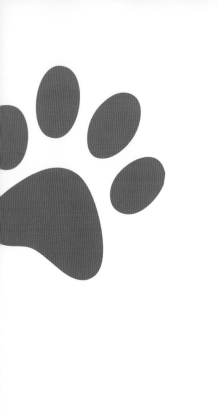

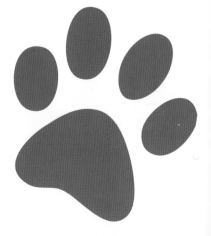

5

Play and attention

Whose toy is that?

Your baby is not the only new arrival in the house that brings new sounds. Even before your baby arrives, toys will start to appear. Some dogs can react quite excitedly or even fearfully to unique toy noises. Other dogs react markedly only to the sound of squeaky toys. This often manifests as barking or howling, which could startle a baby. A track of common baby toy noises (track 12), as well as a track consisting purely of squeaky toys (track 13), is included with this book to accustom your dog to these sounds. Follow through the steps 1 to 3 outlined previously to habituate your dog to these toy sounds, as you replay tracks 12 and 13.

Toys can also be a source of conflict. Baby toys often resemble dog toys, and some people give their dogs old children's toys and dolls. If your dog currently has toys that may resemble your baby's toys (ball, teddy, something squeaky), it is a good idea to discard them. Buy some dog toys that do not resemble baby toys (for example, food-related toys, chew toys and rope toys). Your baby could be unintentionally injured if your dog grabs a toy from their hand.

 Baby toys often resemble dog toys

Distinguish the dog toys from baby toys by rubbing a fragrant herb on the dog toys (for example, mint or rosemary) or spraying a small squirt of unique perfume (not one you use yourself!) onto the toys. You do not need to douse them in scent, as a dog's sense of smell is much more powerful than ours. This smell identifies the toys as your dog's. If your dog orientates towards a baby toy, tell them to 'drop it', reward with a food treat when they do, and then redirect them to their own scented dog toys.

Keep the dog toy box elevated so your dog does not have continual access to all the toys and your child is unable to go exploring through the 'dog only' toy box. Rotate the toys daily or have a toy for each day of the week, so they remain novel and interesting.

There are many varieties of dog toys available. Dog toys are more likely to be played with by your dog if they are associated with food. For recommended toys see **www.babyandpet.com.au**

Somebody notice me!

Attention-seeking behaviour is common in dogs. Jumping up, pawing or forceful nuzzling for attention may currently be endearing behaviours. However, they could be potentially dangerous in the future if they occur while you have your baby in your arms or lap. Other examples of attention-seeking behaviour are mouthing, barking and whining. Whatever the behaviour is, it could be disruptive for a newborn.

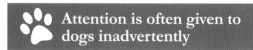

Attention is often given to dogs inadvertently

Your relationship with your dog may need to alter because you will no longer be able to give them attention whenever they demand it. Attention is given to dogs in many ways, often inadvertently. Inadvertent attention includes eye contact and pushing them away with your hands or knees. Even attention that you may think is punishment can be seen as rewarding. For some dogs, for instance, yelling 'no' and 'off' – commands that no longer consistently work. When attention-seeking behaviours that have earned attention in the past are suddenly stopped (for example, when you are busy with your new baby), dogs will often try harder with behaviours that have worked previously, or try new escalated behaviours (for example, barking *and* jumping up) to regain your attention. This is called the frustration effect and could be very disruptive for your new family.

Consistency is the most important factor when (re-)training your dog to stop attention-seeking behaviours. Everyone in the household, including visitors, should adhere to it. Putting a sign on the front door saying, 'Please ignore the dog upon entry' is useful. (Another good one is, 'Shhh! Mum and baby are sleeping.') When your dog demands attention, for example by jumping up, place your hands behind your back and turn your body away from them. Stay silent and do not look at them. If your dog is responsive to simple obedience commands, request them to 'sit' or similar, and if they do respond (and they are no longer jumping up), lavish them with attention (eye contact, treat, pat, stroke, praise, etc.). If they do not respond favourably to your request, do not repeat it, but continue to ignore them and try again later. Remember the frustration effect, described above. The frustration effect is actually a good sign – it indicates that your training is working and the attention-seeking behaviour will soon start to decrease, as long as you continue to be consistent.

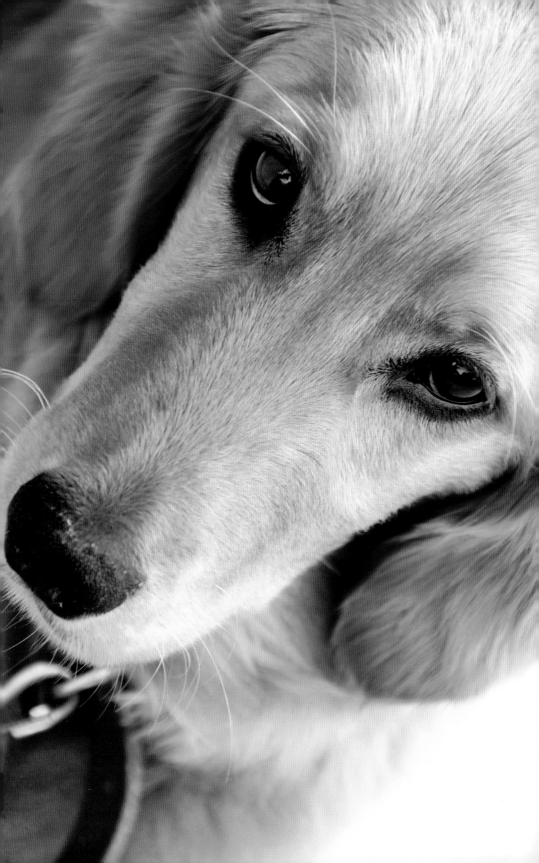

Common attention-seeking problems

Jumping up

If your dog jumps up when you arrive home or when visitors arrive, it could be harmful when you are carrying a baby. The numerous visitors to the new baby may not appreciate it either. Barking at the door when visitors arrive is not always desirable and could also disturb your baby. These specific problems can be caused by a number of things, and may require assistance from a dog trainer.

Mounting or humping

Mounting or humping a person can be seen as humorous (especially if it is your mother-in-law) but it is often an annoying problem. It can be more of an issue if your dog does this to visitors or to you while you are carrying a baby. This type of behaviour is rarely sexual or dominance related, but it may be a sign of your dog's frustration caused by inconsistencies in your interactions with your dog. It may also be attention-seeking.

To stop this behaviour you must first take note of when it occurs. It is likely to be only at certain times or in certain situations. You then need to anticipate when the mounting or humping is likely to occur and direct your dog to a more desirable alternative behaviour *before* it starts.

You need to teach your dog what you would prefer them to do in this situation, other than humping your leg! The alternative behaviour may be to go to their bed and receive a chew toy or it may be to sit next to you and get a food reward and a pat. You need to choose a specific alternative behaviour and always use it to redirect your dog in these situations. This creates more consistent interactions which will assist with your dog's frustration in these circumstances. If it continues to be a problem, seek assistance from an appropriate veterinarian.

Rough play

Rough-housing and play sessions between a dog and their owner can become quite boisterous and involve a lot of noise and sudden fast movements. These interactions should now be restricted to outside, as they could accidentally injure an infant on the floor.

Dog−owner attachments

If your dog is currently highly attached to one particular family member, it would be wise for other members of the family to try and alter this. Less bonded members of the family should take over the fun activities with your dog such as feeding, walking or playing to balance out the attention your dog receives and not have them so reliant on one person. This is especially the case if the most attached person is likely to soon be the most time poor!

 Ensure you have some dedicated one-on-one time with your dog

Time with your dog

Try to ensure you still have some one-on-one time with your dog. This can be both relaxing and enjoyable for parents and dog alike. Have this time equally when the baby is present and also when the baby is asleep or absent. This will mean your dog will not associate the baby's presence with a negative feeling of being ignored.

An important adjunct to ignoring unwanted attention-seeking behaviours is to reward your dog when they are showing desirable behaviours. Throw them a tasty treat when they are relaxed on their bed; call them over for a loving pat when they are resting; or calmly tell them they are a 'good dog' while they are chewing on a dog toy.

This is great practice for future parenting too!

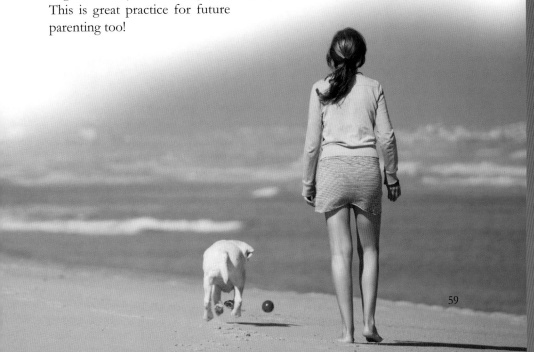

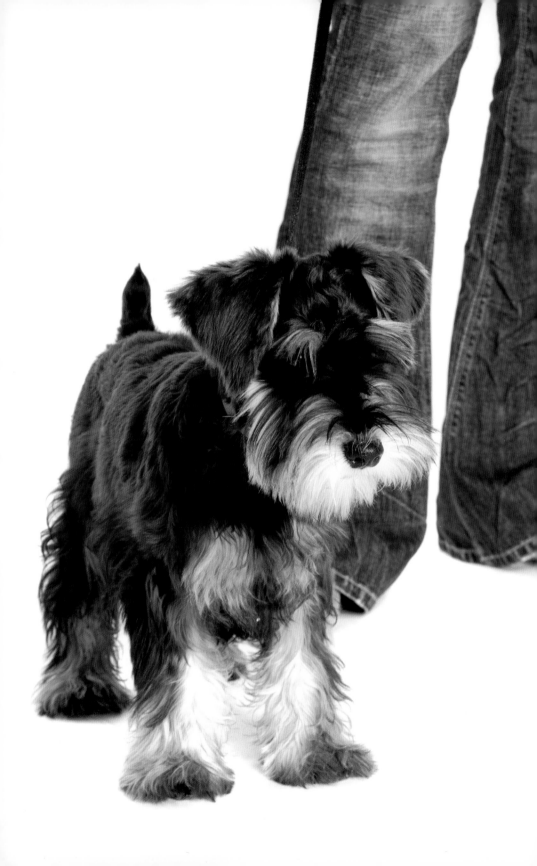

Case study: The furry leg warmer

When I first entered Jane and Greg's house I didn't need to be told what the problem was with Charlie, a three-year-old desexed male Schnauzer. For the first twenty minutes after I walked in the front door, Charlie proceeded to 'make love' to my leg. He did stop for a minute when I sat on the couch and then he switched to humping and mounting my other leg. It made for an hilarious but slightly embarrassing consultation. For health and safety reasons, I declined the offered cup of hot coffee and despite the adoration of my new-found friend I proceeded to listen to Jane and Greg's story.

Jane and Greg were expecting their first child later that year and they were concerned Charlie's humping was getting out of control. Charlie would hump both Jane and Greg with great excitement when they arrived home and also when they tried to tell him off for misbehaving. He would also mount visitors and occasionally his favourite soft toy. Jane was rightly concerned that Charlie might push her over when she was carrying the baby but also that there would be more visitors to the house who would not enjoy his 'advances'. The humping had been escalating for over two years and various techniques to control the problem had been recommended, but it seemed that every technique they tried just made it worse.

After discussing (and watching) Jane and Greg's interactions with Charlie it became apparent that they were often inconsistent. Sometimes when Charlie pawed one of them for attention they would give it to him, but at other times they would tell him 'no' and push him away. When he greeted them excitedly at the door Jane and Greg would sometimes give him big cuddles but at other times tell him 'off' or 'down'. Poor Charlie was terribly confused. He didn't know how to interact correctly with his owners to get a favourable response.

I recommended to Jane and Greg they re-introduce some basic obedience into the house. They were also only to reward Charlie when he was displaying appropriate quiet behaviour such as sitting or lying on his mat, and to ignore unwanted behaviour such us jumping up or humping. When interacting with Charlie, they were to use structured interactions where they requested a specific behaviour from Charlie (for example, sitting) and when he performed that behaviour, he would be rewarded.

When I visited Jane and Greg some six months later, I braced myself for the furry leg greeting as the front door opened. Instead, I was greeted pleasantly by a heavily pregnant Jane with Charlie sitting next to her with his tail wagging excitedly – no more leg cuddles! Needless to say Charlie was a changed man.

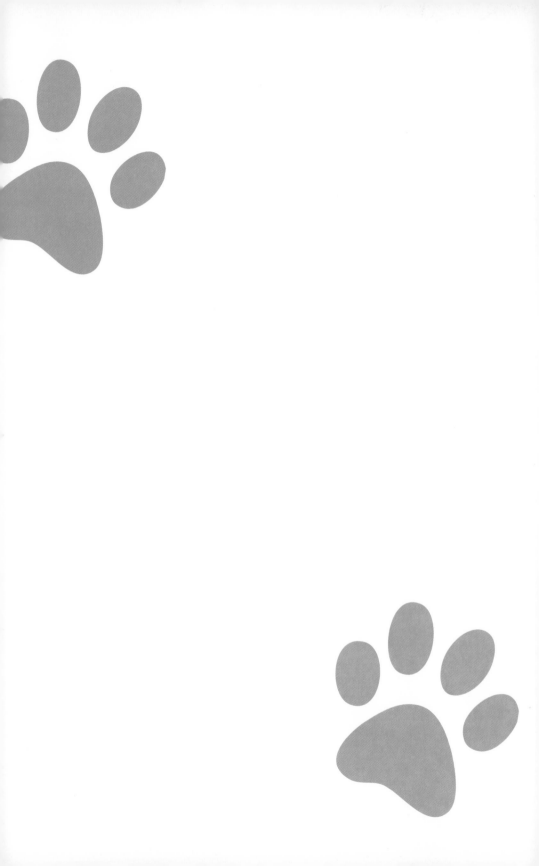

6

Routines

Be predictable and consistent

With the arrival of a baby, routines, consistency and predictable (good) interactions often go out the window. These changes can make a dog unsure or anxious in the home and lead to problems. Interacting with your dog in a consistent, predictable manner where your dog can be sure of receiving a good outcome (that is, a treat or praise), can greatly assist in reducing the anxiety associated with these changes.

To create this predictability and consistency, you may have to change your current interactions with your dog. All members of the household must behave consistently and make the change. If only one person alters the way they interact with your dog and others do not, your dog will not gain the predictability that this training brings. Unthinking or random interactions with your dog contribute to an unpredictable environment and should therefore be avoided. Future interactions should be highly structured using this sequence:

1. Ask your dog to do something (for example, sit or drop).
2. Your dog responds favourably (that is, sits or drops).
3. Your dog is rewarded (for example, food, pat or attention).

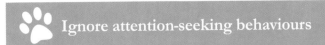 Ignore attention-seeking behaviours

As outlined previously, attention-seeking behaviours should be ignored. Rewards and attention should only be given when your dog responds favourably to your requests. It can be difficult to ignore your dog when they do solicit attention, but this aspect of behaviour modification is quite important if you want to teach your dog to be more independent. Increasing the predictability of your day-to-day interactions with your dog can help to alleviate anxiety. It also provides your dog with some control over their environment, in that they now know that to receive something favourable they must behave in a desirable way.

Your dog and schedules

Before your baby is born, introduce a regular schedule that you will realistically be able to adhere to when your baby arrives. Start with play, walking and feeding schedules. But do not be fooled! A new baby requires an extraordinary amount of time.

When you think about feeding a newborn up to eight times a day, and remember that this can take an hour each time, you begin to understand how your time disappears, especially when each feed results in a nappy change. As well as tending to your new baby, you will be faced with a plethora of chores that need to be performed, not to mention allowing time to just hold, gaze at, cuddle and enjoy your new baby! There will also be extra visitors to see you and your new baby, and they take up further time. All this will be radically different from your current routine. It is unlikely that you will have time to walk your dog for an hour, or play fetch for long periods when your baby requires three-hourly (or more frequent) feeds and several sleeps during the day.

Gradually decrease the interaction time with your dog over several months to a level that you honestly believe you will be able to manage when your baby arrives. To keep the bond with your dog strong, dedicate a minimum period (for example, ten minutes) twice daily to focusing exclusively on your dog. The most appropriate time for this may be when another person is available to monitor your baby, allowing you to give your dog your full attention. During this time, talk to them, pat them, groom them and play with their toys. Try hard to maintain this schedule and make it one that can be easily done when your baby arrives home. Ideally, set a (quiet) alarm or reminder so as not to miss your dog's special time.

 Don't miss out on your dog's special time!

'Walkies' time!

Dogs should ideally be walked twice daily to provide adequate mental and physical stimulation. This does vary with temperament, breed and age. New parents and baby also benefit from the fresh air and exercise! The more often you exercise your dog with your baby, the better their relationship is likely to be.

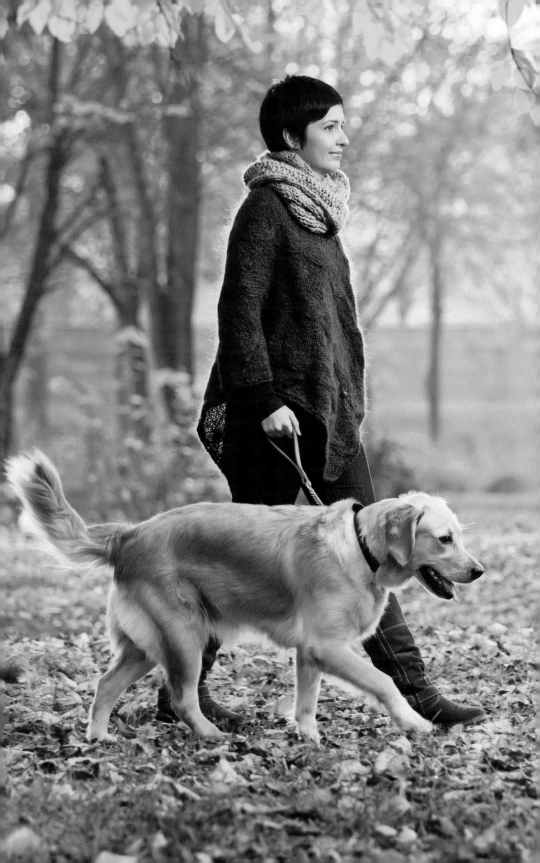

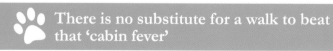

Regular walking

Begin a walking schedule for your dog that you can maintain when your baby arrives. Make this realistic and not always at a specific set time during the day.

If regular walking is likely to be a problem, employ a dog walker or, better still, make use of willing friends, family or neighbours to walk your dog. Consider the use of dog day-care facilities to provide your dog with mental and physical stimulation. Ensure that you visit the facility and give your dog a trial run before your baby arrives. Sometimes a simple exercise like throwing the ball for ten minutes in the backyard can provide some much-needed physical stimulation for your dog. Be aware that there is no substitute for a good walk to beat that 'cabin fever'.

Prams

Incorporate your new pram into your dog walks several weeks before your baby arrives. This will assist you to gauge your dog's response to the pram – some dogs are unaccustomed to moving objects with wheels, and many prams and strollers squeak, bounce and rattle. You can also assess your ability to control both your dog and the pram at the same time. Ideally, you want to be able to walk with your dog and the pram together and not run the risk of being injured or pulled off course. Many dogs get quite excited at the sight of the pram, as it means walk time. If your dog pulls on the lead or you do not have

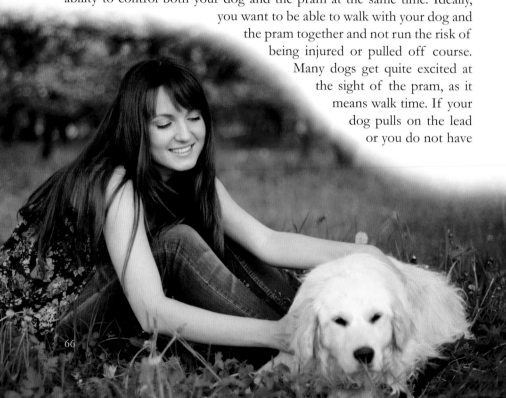

66

good control, consider purchasing a head collar or non-pulling harness (see **www.babyandpet.com.au**), or seek assistance from a dog trainer.

Regardless of your dog's size or temperament, never tie them to your pram, especially when your pram is 'parked'. It does not take much pulling power to tip over a pram or roll the pram into a dangerous situation.

Slings and backpacks

If you plan to use a sling, carrier, front or backpack, start carrying your pretend baby (see step 5 earlier) around in it to become accustomed to controlling your dog with something else attached to you.

Dog fights

If your dog is aggressive or uncontrollable towards other dogs this is a potentially dangerous situation. If you or your baby become entangled in a fight between dogs, one or both of you can easily get bitten or injured. So if your dog displays this behaviour you need to seek assistance from an appropriate veterinarian.

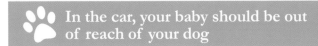

In the car, your baby should be out of reach of your dog

Car travelling

An unrestrained dog inside a car is undesirable and dangerous for you and your baby, so ensure your dog is adequately restrained well before you install your car baby capsule. Confine your dog in the back section of a station wagon, buy a seatbelt harness, or train your dog to accept car travel in a dog carrier or crate. Your baby should be out of reach of your dog at all times in the car. If your dog currently has problems with vomiting, drooling, barking, howling or is unable to settle in the car, you may want to seek assistance from an appropriate veterinarian. You may like to practise specific difficult activities well before your baby arrives, for example, entering and leaving the house or strapping your pretend baby and dog into their respective car seats.

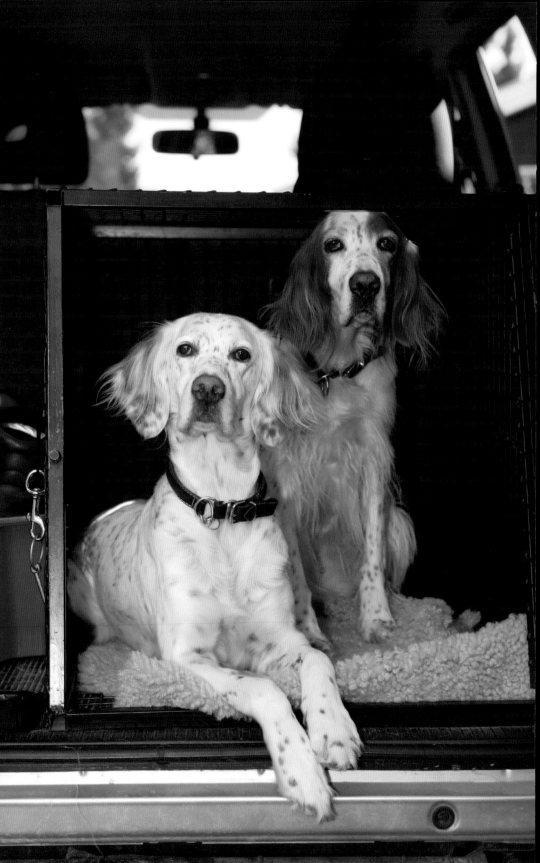

Your dog and touch

Start training your dog to accept child-like touching all over their body. This process is called desensitisation. Some dogs are sensitive to having particular areas touched, for example, their feet or tail. When touched in certain areas these dogs may show signs outlined in behaviour groups B or C. Even if your dog does not display these signs it can be wise to get them used to being touched, because young children grab whatever is going past.

Desensitise your dog by touching them lightly all over, and offering food or play as rewards for not reacting unfavourably. Do this slowly and calmly, ensuring that your dog is relaxed at all times. If your dog reacts to touch of a certain kind, then move to patting a less-sensitive area and slowly work back to the upsetting area with a much lighter touch. Start by touching favourite areas, for example, the head, and move slowly to less enjoyable areas, for example, the feet. Gradually, over a period of time, increase the pressure of your touches while continuing with these rewards. Areas to focus on are feet, ears, tail, collar and fur tugging.

After a period of training, and if your dog responds well to controlled slow touches and fur tugs, then start making fast random movements towards different parts of their body and giving them a heavy pat or a fur tug. Reward them instantly with a treat for displaying a relaxed response. Do this at different times of the day and in different situations. Your dog will then learn to associate touching and fur tugging with good things like a treat, rather than perceiving them as unfavourable.

These training exercises are intended to mimic the sudden movements of a young child grasping your dog. They will *never guarantee* that your dog will not react to a tail grab or fur tug from a child, for example, but it may mean that your dog will not be as reactive as they are currently. These exercises do not remove the need for constant adult supervision of your dog and child.

Some dogs may not respond well to this training and will not tolerate certain areas of their body being touched. If the process described above does not seem to be reducing the intensity of your dog's reaction, then this is potentially an area of conflict between your dog and your baby. You may need to seek assistance from an appropriate veterinarian.

Who's hungry?

Currently you may be feeding your dog elaborately-cooked meals. You may not be able to maintain this with your new routine. Consider discussing with your veterinarian a suitable, more convenient food. It's a good idea to buy enough dog food and treats before the baby's arrival to ensure an adequate supply.

Gradually decrease the rigidity of the actual feeding time, so your dog does not expect their food at exactly the same time each day. If your dog begs for food or snatches food off the dinner table or from hands, you should place them in a separate area or train them to go to a specific area at meal times.

Ideally, adult dogs should be fed twice daily in a separate, safe and secure area. Food should not be available 24/7 and any food remaining after 20 to 30 minutes should be removed.

Resource guarding

Some dogs are (aggressively) protective of their food, bones, rawhides, treats or chews. This is called 'resource guarding' and can also apply to items such as toys or other possessions. A dog that is a resource guarder will show one or several of the signs outlined in behaviour groups B or C when approached while in possession of one or more of these items. This

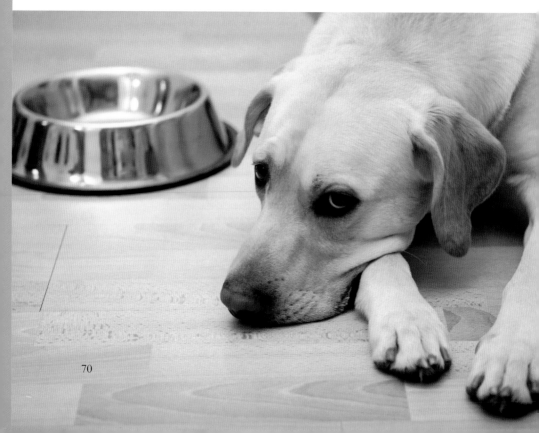

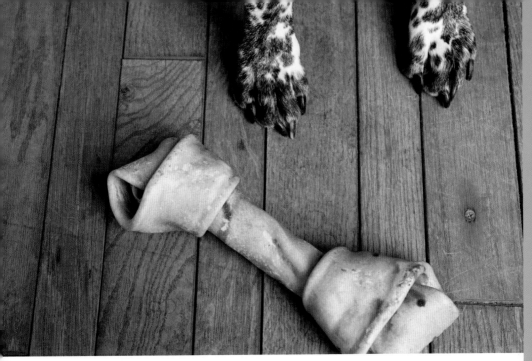

problem needs to be addressed urgently as a recent scientific study highlighted that 61 per cent of dogs that had a history of biting children were resource guarders.

If the resource guarding *only* occurs when your dog is in possession of *one type of dog-specific* item and nothing else (for example, *only* bones or *only* rawhide chews) then either excluding these (that is, bones or rawhide chews) from your dog's life or only giving them in a safe, secure area are the safest options. Your dog should only be allowed out of the safe secure area when the item is finished or your dog has moved away from the item and it can be safely removed (that is, placed out of the dog's reach).

 ## Generalised resource guarding is a serious problem

If the resource guarding occurs when your dog is in possession of one type of *non*-dog-specific item (for example, squeaky toys) or is more generalised and extends to daily meals, treats, rawhides, chews, bones or toys, then this is a more complex problem to manage. Your dog is guarding items that are *not only dog-specific* items but rather items that they will encounter every day in a family home. For instance, babies will accidentally drop food from the highchair; or a crawling child holding food or a toy could easily approach your dog. It is not suitable to just 'feed your resource-guarding dog separately', as this generalised resource guarding is more serious and needs to be addressed now by consulting an appropriate veterinarian.

Taking precautions

Even if your dog is *not* currently a resource guarder, this is one type of aggression that occasionally appears when a new baby is brought home. It is wise to take precautions against this now, rather than being sorry later.

In anticipation that your dog *may* develop resource guarding, start implementing some simple exercises before the baby arrives, to reward your dog for appropriate behaviour when approached while they are eating or in possession of a valued item (for example, a bone or toy). While your dog is engaged with an item, randomly drop some very tasty food rewards into the bowl or next to them as you walk past. Only do this if your dog shows none of the signs outlined in behaviour groups B or C when you approach. In this way you are rewarding them for behaving appropriately when someone goes near them when they have possession of an item. This exercise *does not* replace the ideal situation of your dog being fed in a separate, safe and secure area, but it may help to decrease the chance of your dog reacting unfavourably (for the first time) if accidentally approached by a child while eating.

Water bowls

These should be slightly elevated or in a separate area out of reach of babies. Changing your dog's water bowl to a flat, shallow bowl may prevent accidental drowning.

Rewards and treats

Place several containers filled with small treats around the house out of your dog's reach. They should be only accessible to adults. This will enable you to instantly reward your dog for appropriate behaviour without missing an opportunity. A reward or treat only needs to be the size of a large crumb to effectively convey the message.

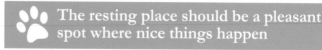

The resting place should be a pleasant spot where nice things happen

Time for a rest

Create an area where your dog can safely retreat for some 'me time' and not be disturbed. This could also be an area that your dog will go to when asked. It may be an enclosed area that your dog can jump into, or a crate, or a dedicated blanket or mat. It should be an area separate from your baby, where your dog cannot be cornered by a crawling child (for example, not a couch where a toddler could pull themselves up and block the escape route).

Ensure that your dog is comfortable being separated from you in such an area before your baby arrives. When separated from their owner, some dogs can become destructive, bark or howl, urinate or defecate. If this is your dog, you need to slowly train them to go to this area by throwing small treats, feeding meals and giving attention and food rewards when they are in this area. Never use it as a punishment area, but rather make it a pleasant place where nice things happen.

Currently your dog may be enjoying the comfort of the couch or similar piece of furniture to relax. This is not a problem as long as your dog can be easily moved or disturbed without showing adverse signs (behaviour groups B or C). If your dog is showing these signs, a simple solution may be to not allow your dog onto these areas anymore. It may be preferable to

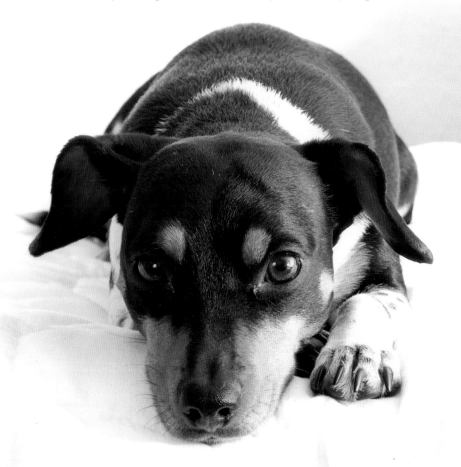

train your dog to jump onto the couch only when invited. This invitation may be a particular word you use, or even a uniquely patterned blanket that is laid down when your dog is allowed to get on the couch. This decision needs to be made early and training must start before your baby arrives. If this adverse behaviour is widespread for many resting areas, seek assistance from an appropriate veterinarian.

Can my dog sleep on my bed?

Many owners ask, 'Is it okay for my dog to sleep on my bed?' A dog sleeping on their owner's bed is usually only a problem if your dog reacts unfavourably (behaviour groups B or C) when you are in bed or when you try to remove them from the bed. If this is your dog, then sleeping or resting on the bed should not be allowed. You need to start training your dog to sleep elsewhere. This should not be a place where you will stumble over them during the night when rushing to your baby.

If you are planning for your baby to sleep in bed with you (consult your paediatrician regarding current SIDS guidelines), or you are planning to give some feeds in bed, your dog should not be sleeping in your bed or even in your bedroom. While you are asleep or just dozing (as mothers often do when feeding), it is not possible to monitor interactions between your dog and your baby. It is not uncommon for a dog to surreptitiously crawl into bed with exhausted parents!

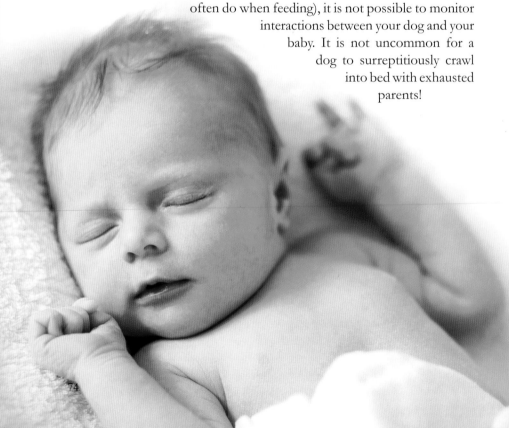

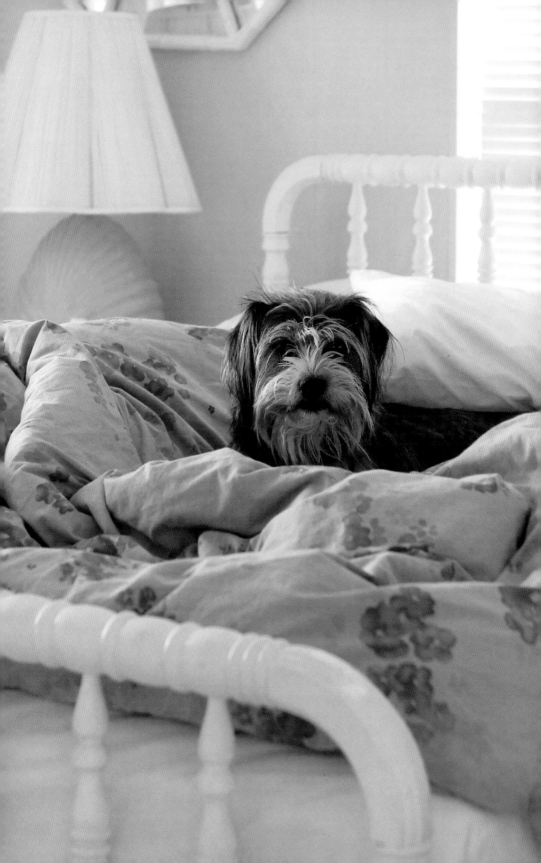

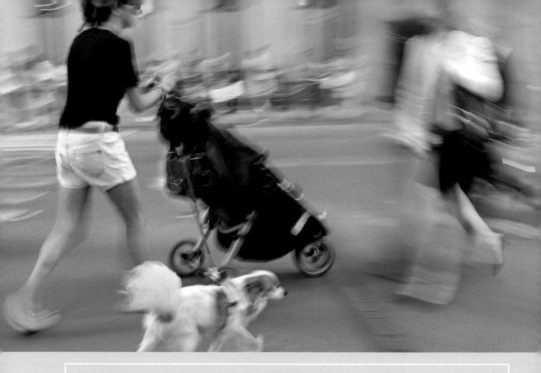

Case study 1: Dreams vs reality

Claire rang me in urgent need of help with her dog, Jeeves, a five-year-old Blue Heeler. Claire was five months pregnant and had visions of walking contentedly with her baby in the pram with Jeeves trotting along by her side. This dream was shattered each time she walked Jeeves. He pulled on the lead, he whined and barked at loud trucks or buses and he didn't always come when he was called. All of these traits were simply not conducive to happy family walks. Claire needed to be able to walk Jeeves safely on the lead while wheeling a pram. She had some work to do!

Claire was aware that Jeeves was a very energetic dog who needed lots of mental stimulation and exercise. Thankfully, she was committed to walking Jeeves daily, both before and after the arrival of her new baby. Jeeves was trained to accept a head halter to minimise pulling on the lead. We also began training Jeeves, using food rewards and praise, to reliably sit on command inside the house. This was then extended to sit commands during the walk and then also when loud trucks approached. This enabled him to start enjoying the approach of a loud vehicle because he knew he should sit and then he would get a tasty food reward. Once Claire felt comfortable, we then introduced her flashy new pram to the walks and reinforced Jeeves's good behaviour with rewards.

Jeeves responded exceptionally well to the adjustments made to his walks. He still doesn't always come when he is called – that is a work in progress – but Claire's dreams of walks with her new baby and dog have become a reality.

Case study 2: A difficult situation

Jill and Paul asked me to visit them and their dog, Kaya, a two-year-old medium-sized crossbred. She was showing signs of aggression and this had increased markedly since the arrival of their new baby, Sophia.

For the last twelve months, when Kaya was resting in certain places, she had been growling whenever Jill or Paul approached. Initially it was just one spot on the couch but now, since Sophia had arrived, it was several places, including both of the couches and her bed. If either of them tried to move her she would snap at them. Paul was nursing a couple of stitches in his arm from where Kaya had bitten him the previous week.

On further discussion, I discovered Kaya was also aggressive when she was in possession of bones and certain dog toys. Jill had also noticed that Kaya would freeze and stare at her if she approached while the dog was eating from her bowl.

Jill and Paul were now scared of Kaya and had adjusted their whole living arrangements to accommodate Kaya's aggression. They had even bought Kaya her very own sofa but she just ended up guarding this new one as well as the original couch! Now they were scared for the safety of their new baby, Sophia, and needed help.

I explained to Jill and Paul that Kaya had a condition called 'resource guarding'. Kaya, for whatever reason, felt uncomfortable when someone approached her if she was in possession of a highly valued item or resting in a comfortable place. Resource guarding is a complex problem and I was very concerned about having a new baby in this environment.

Jill and Paul asked my opinion. I felt it was highly likely that Kaya would injure somebody again in the future. Had their household not contained a new baby, I felt that we could have worked with Kaya and managed, but never cured, this aggression. With the arrival of Sophia, however, the risk was too great and I told them that, in my opinion, Kaya should be euthanased. Given the stitches in Paul's arm, I felt it was too dangerous to try to find her a new home. I left Jill and Paul's home feeling upset about the decision they had to make.

Ten days later, Paul rang to thank me. They had put Kaya to sleep earlier that week. Paul was understandably devastated but also mentioned that his and Jill's stress levels were a lot lower. They had not realised how much energy they had been using tip-toeing around Kaya and her resource guarding. I was terribly saddened by the loss of Kaya but I was comforted by the knowledge that I had avoided their baby, Sophia, becoming a dog-bite statistic.

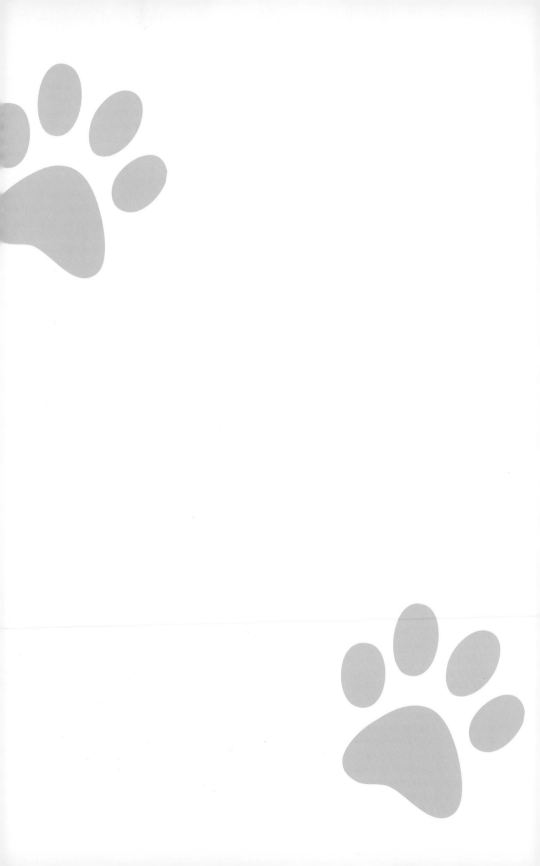

7

Staying healthy

To keep everyone healthy, first make sure your baby, your dog and your house are kept clean. Second, attend to any health issues immediately.

Basic preventative health care

- Ensure your dog is regularly examined by your veterinarian and is up to date with their vaccinations. Most veterinarians recommend a health check every 6 to 12 months.
- Treat your dog regularly for internal parasites (for example, intestinal worms) and external parasites (for example, fleas, ticks and mites) as some are transmissible to humans. Consult your veterinarian for the products most suitable for your dog and your geographical location. Buy an adequate supply in advance.
- Clean up dog faeces regularly. Babies have less resistance than adults to certain causes of gastroenteritis and other diseases caught from faeces.
- Dog bedding should be regularly washed and carpets vacuumed.
- Keep your dog's nails trimmed short to avoid accidental scratching.
- Make a regular booking with your local dog groomer to keep your dog's coat clean and free of tangles. This is more important if your dog has a long coat; keep it clipped short and neat.
- It is recommended to have your dog desexed to decrease the likelihood of health problems to do with the reproductive system. There is some evidence that desexed dogs are less reactive or aggressive.

Medical conditions

- If your dog develops any skin conditions or gastrointestinal problems, have them examined immediately by a veterinarian, as some of these are contagious for humans. Similarly, if there are skin conditions or gastrointestinal conditions among family members, have your dog examined.

- Any current or undiagnosed medical conditions can cause a dog to have a lower threshold of tolerance to changes in their environment. These are more common in older dogs but can occur in younger dogs too. Some specific problems are arthritis, lameness, teeth problems, ear infections, anal gland problems and skin conditions. In one scientific study, 50 per cent of dogs that had bitten children also had concurrent skin or bone issues. For this reason, it is advisable for your dog to have a complete veterinary examination soon after your pregnancy is confirmed so that any potential problems can be rectified early. Regular blood tests may also be recommended by your veterinarian.

Medications and pheromones

- All dog medications should be stored in a child-proof cabinet.
- Dog Appeasing Pheromone (DAP/ADAPTIL) is a product that can be bought from your veterinarian. It is a synthetic canine pheromone, a copy of a substance that is naturally produced by the female dog when she is lactating. It can have a relaxing effect on some dogs in potentially stressful situations, such as introducing a new baby, regardless of the dog's age or sex. It comes in three forms – plug-in diffuser, collar and spray. The plug-in diffuser covers 50 to 70 square metres (540 to 750 square feet) and should be placed in the main room in the house. In addition or alternatively, you may choose to fit a pheromone collar to your dog. Start using one or more of these forms approximately two weeks before your due date. The spray form can be used to assist with the introductions when you first bring the baby home. Spray it onto your clothes and allow it to dry. It is not recommended to spray it directly onto skin or your baby's clothes. DAP/ADAPTIL products are not available in all countries so check with your veterinarian or see **www.babyandpet.com.au** for more information.
- Aromatherapy with lavender or chamomile may assist with a calm first meeting between your dog and your baby.
- Some dogs may benefit from anti-anxiety medication to assist with the initial stress of the appearance of a newborn. Many of these medications do not show results instantly, but need time to achieve the desired effect. These medications are only available on prescription from your veterinarian.

Family hygiene

- Ensure that all family members wash their hands before meal-times, after cleaning the yard, playing outside or touching your dog.
- All nappy buckets should have a firm, sealable lid to prevent their use as a dog drinking bowl. Ensure they will not accidentally open, even when filled with water, tipped on their side and rolled around.
- Soiled disposable nappies should be placed in bins not accessible to your dog.
- Do not allow your dog to lick your baby's face. This can be dangerous, not only from a behaviour perspective but also because some worms can be spread in this manner. If your dog does lick your baby's face or licks other areas of your baby (for example, feet), normal preventative hygiene should apply.
- If your baby is unwell or you are concerned about their health then contact your doctor or physician.

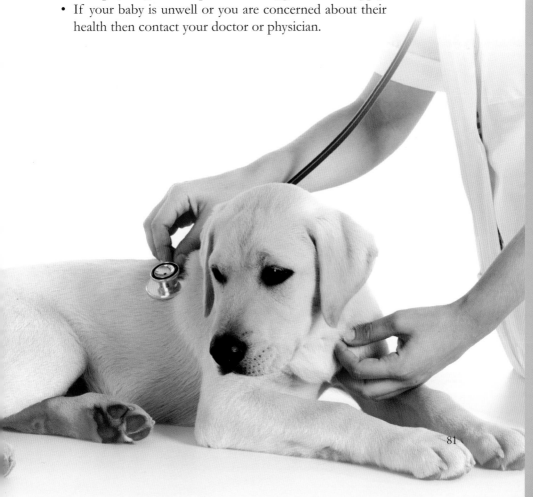

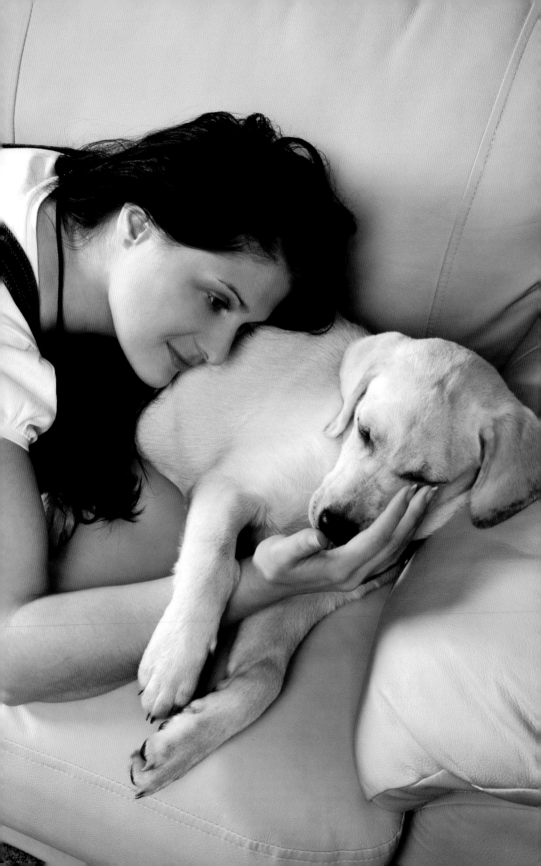

Case study: I can't walk, my ear hurts!

Caroline brought Missy, a six-year-old Australian Shepherd, into the veterinary clinic for her yearly health check. She mentioned that Missy had been reasonably well but in the last week had refused to go on her usual walk. Caroline had recently given birth to a gorgeous baby boy, Zac, and she assumed that Missy did not want to go for walks because she was upset about sharing her walks with Zac riding in his pram. She needed some advice.

While we were chatting, I gave Missy a clinical examination to make sure she was healthy. When I tried to look in her left ear she cowered away from me and rubbed at her ear with her paw. With some assistance from a nurse I was able to look down Missy's ear. After some tests it was discovered that she had an ear infection. I suspected that this may have been the cause of her reluctance to go on walks.

When I suggested this to Caroline she then remembered that Missy didn't want to go for a run with her husband, Sam, on the weekend and this was also unusual. Sam did not take the pram. I suggested we start treating the ear condition with medication and then monitor Missy's behaviour over the next week.

Ten days later Caroline (and Missy) returned with a big smile. Missy had regained her normal enthusiasm for her walks and runs. This had occurred about four days after commencement of the ear medication. Caroline thought it was a miracle and was very happy that Missy now happily trotted next to the pram. A quick examination of her ear showed that it was free from infection.

Problems that coincide with a new baby coming into the family may have other causes, so a health check is always a good idea. Who would have thought a sore ear could stop a dog enjoying their walks!

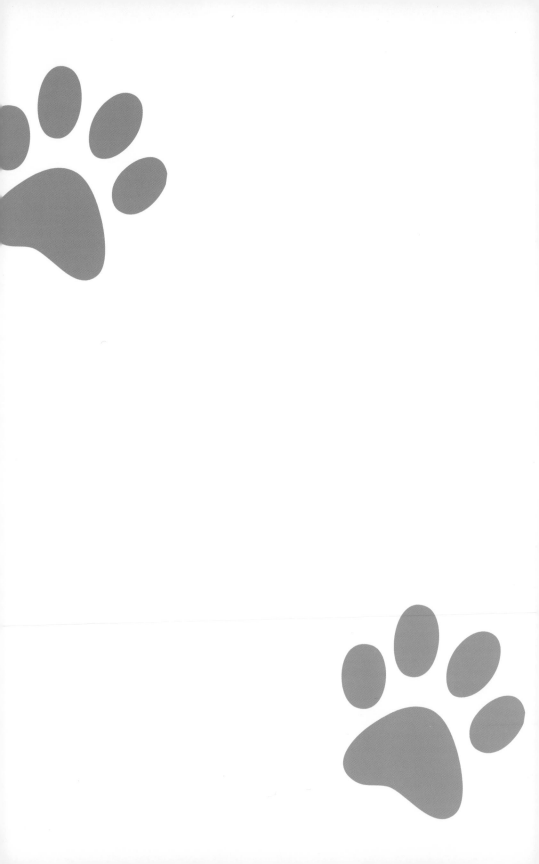

8

Are you ready?

Preparing the nursery

Familiarising your dog

- Introduce your dog to the new baby items before the baby is born. This includes: the cot or crib, change table, baby rocker, high chair, bouncer, pram, play mat, nappies, nappy-rash creams and powders, shampoos and soaps, blankets and toys. Also include any other new furniture or items in the house. Do not be concerned that your dog may put hair or dirt on these things. Allow your dog to smell and investigate them. Reward your dog for correct behaviour. If your dog drags any baby items away, use the 'drop it' command to ask your dog to relinquish the object and then replace it with a dog toy or treat. Try not to punish your dog, as you want only good things occurring with anything associated with your baby.

 Reward your dog for desirable behaviour

- Place your pretend baby in each of these items and perform the activities you are likely to do with your baby while considering where you would like your dog to be at this time.
- Have periods of relaxation in the nursery with your dog, allowing them to investigate the nursery while supervised. This could be accompanied by a favourite food-filled toy, chew or bone.
- Do not leave baby items lying around and easily accessible in case your dog becomes destructive with them.

Furniture and equipment

- A special mention needs to be made of motorised baby swings. There have been documented cases in the United States of babies being harmed or killed by dogs while in a motorised swing. As always, babies and dogs should be supervised at all times. Never leave your baby in a motorised swing where your dog has access. Safely and securely separate them. Before your baby arrives, prepare your dog by placing your pretend baby in the swing and turning it on at the slowest and quietest setting to gauge your dog's response. Follow steps 2 to 5 as outlined previously while monitoring your dog's behaviour using the behaviour groups. Even after following these steps you should still supervise or separate your baby and dog when using a swing.

- Your dog should not sleep on or near any of your baby's furniture. Block off access to the nursery when you are not present to stop your dog from resting in this area.
- Buy a baby monitor, even if your baby is always going to be near you, as it can give extra security by ensuring there are no inadvertent visitors in your baby's room.
- Buy a cordless home telephone so you do not have to leave your dog and baby when answering a phone call.

While you are in hospital

Who's looking after me?

Organise early on for somebody to 'dog-sit' your dog in your own home while you are in the hospital or birthing centre. It should preferably be someone your dog knows well. Boarding your dog or moving them to another house is a less suitable option as there may be associated anxiety, particularly when they arrive back home to a totally changed environment. However, if this is necessary, have a trial run to ensure you and your dog feel comfortable with the arrangement. This allows your dog to become acquainted with the people and environment where they will be staying, which can make their stay less stressful.

Can I come too?

Expectant parents may feel that they would like their 'first baby' to be present when their human baby arrives. It is not recommended that your dog is present at the baby's birth. Birthing is often a stressful experience for both the mother and the newborn. Dogs intuitively pick up on this stress. It is counter-productive for the first introduction to be in such an emotional setting, and this goes against the philosophy of associating good things with the baby.

Case study: A smelly problem

I received a phone call from Sally who insisted that I see her and Buster as soon as possible. Buster was a six-year-old Boxer cross. Sally told me that she adored Buster and that he was a lovely dog with an even temperament and had been very gentle with Sally's new baby, Lachlan. After juggling some appointments I went to see them the next day.

When I arrived at Sally's house, Buster was outside and he greeted me at the side gate. He did indeed appear to be a lovely dog. After greeting Sally and tiptoeing down the hall past Lachlan, who was sleeping peacefully in his crib, I soon smelt and then noticed the problem. On the corners of the door-ways and the legs of the sofas I noticed the tell-tale signs of urine marks. Buster had clearly been very busy and I could see and smell why Sally needed urgent help.

Sally was a single mum who had recently moved back into her parents' house. Lachlan had arrived prematurely and so the house move coincided with his arrival. Buster had previously been an indoor dog when Sally was living on her own. The problem was that whenever Buster was let inside her parents' house and not monitored, he would urine mark. Now he had been banished to the backyard and the laundry at night. Sally wanted him back inside as part of the family as soon as possible.

Buster clearly was not coping with so many changes to his routine and environment in such a short space of time. I discussed with Sally strategies to help Buster cope with all these changes. We discussed how to clean up the urine to make the area less attractive for Buster the next time. As Buster was a complex case, and Sally was a busy single mum, I also prescribed medication and pheromones for Buster.

After several emails over a period of eighteen months, I decided it was time to revisit Buster. When I arrived this time Buster was not at the side gate. As Sally opened the front door I was pleasantly surprised to be greeted by Buster inside the house. Following Buster was Lachlan, walking unsteadily down the hallway with arms outstretched for a cuddle. At this point my heart sank; there was a new smell in the house – poo. Did Buster have a new problem? Sally must have noticed the look on my face as she scooped up Lachlan and took him off to change his poo-filled nappy. Having two children of my own, it was the first time I can remember being pleased to smell a dirty nappy rather than dog urine!

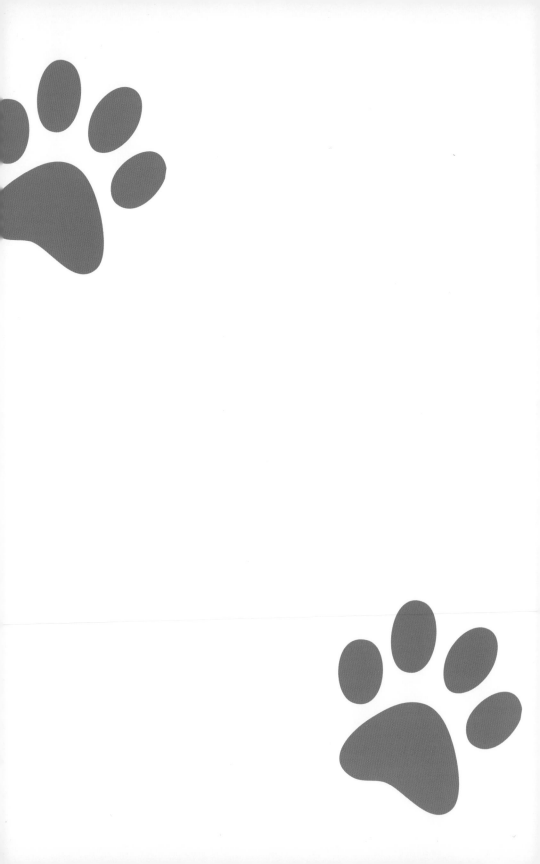

9

Your baby is born!

Congratulations! You are now proud parents! Currently, Mum is still in hospital with the baby. Her partner now has some important tasks to perform to prepare the dog at home.

The newborn smell

Smell is one of a dog's most important senses. They have an incredible sense of smell which is much better than that of humans. For this reason, your partner needs to bring home some of the following items to start introducing your baby to the dog: a soiled nappy, something that your baby has worn (for example, a jumpsuit, singlet, muslin wrap or blanket), a used breast pad and a used pacifier or bottle teat (if your baby uses these). These all contain important olfactory cues enabling your dog to become acquainted with your baby even before they arrive home. Allow your dog to sniff the objects, and reward them lavishly with treats and pats for correct behaviour. If they start to become overly interested in the item (for example, chewing or pawing) then distract your dog and reward them for performing a different behaviour (for example, sitting or coming for a pat). Do not leave these items lying around unsupervised. Wrap the pretend baby in a blanket or clothing that your newborn baby has worn, and perform a couple of sessions with the tracks in the specific locations, as outlined earlier in steps 4 and 5. At the same time, talk to your dog in an upbeat voice, telling them about the new arrival and using your baby's name.

Meeting the baby

You now have your dog prepared in the best way possible for your impending arrival. They know what sounds to expect (via the CD), they know what the little person smells like and they have adapted to the new household routine. Now it is time to meet the family!

The day your baby is due to arrive home, have someone take your dog for a walk a couple of hours before you arrive, to tire them slightly. Allow at least 20 minutes between the end of the walk and your arrival so that your dog is not still overly exuberant from their walk. Most dogs get very excited when the walking leash is brought out and attached to their collar because it means they are about to go for a walk (even if they have just been for one!). For this reason, ask the walker to leave the leash and collar, head collar or harness on your dog after they have been walked so that you do not need to re-attach these when you arrive home. Do not leave your dog unsupervised with a leash attached to their collar, head collar or harness as they could accidentally harm themselves.

Limit the number of people present at the first meeting

Limit the number of people present at the first meeting. When Mum first arrives home from hospital your dog will be very excited to see her again. They will also be excited to see her partner, who may have been away too. An excited dog greeting you and your new baby for the first time is likely to end in problems. Have someone, other than you or your partner, cuddle your baby outside the house while you both go in and greet your dog. In this way, you can give them your full attention without worrying about them hurting your baby. Once your dog is calm, introductions can begin.

The most important thing to remember when your dog meets your baby is that good things should always happen to your dog whenever your baby is around. Whenever your baby is present, give your dog tasty food rewards and loads of praise.

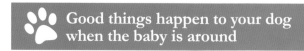

Good things happen to your dog when the baby is around

One partner should sit comfortably on a chair at a table as if they are going to eat a meal. Your baby should be in their lap. This enables easy control of the amount of access your dog initially has to your baby. The other partner should monitor and have full control of your dog. Use a leash with a fixed length attached to a collar, head collar or harness. Both parents need to take a deep breath and try to relax for this introduction. If you are visibly anxious or distressed, your dog will sense this. Talk gently to your dog while patting and stroking them. Under strict supervision, encourage them to smell and investigate your baby. Reward them for appropriate behaviour with food rewards or pats and an up-beat, calm voice.

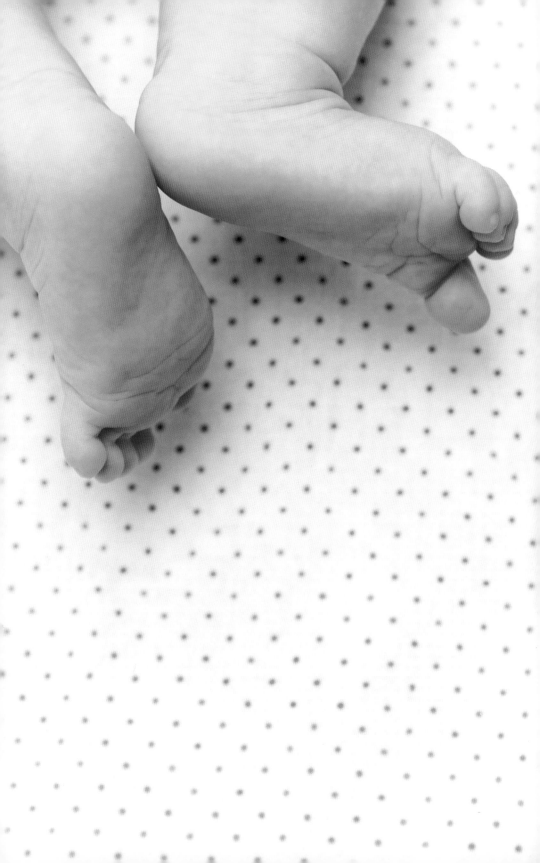

Remember to take it very slowly. Do not rush the meeting – they have a lifetime to be friends. Do not force your dog to interact if they do not appear to want to, and do not hold or dangle the child in front of your dog. Be pleased if your dog is ambivalent, relaxed or slightly attentive (behaviour group A) in your baby's presence – this is desirable.

 Take it slowly and don't rush the first meeting – they have a lifetime to be friends

Meeting problems

If your dog becomes too excited, tries to jump up at your baby or tries to get between you and your baby, distract them away with food or play and separate them until they settle. Then try again. If your dog shows signs outlined in behaviour groups B or C, then they may be unsure about your baby. Try again at a later time, this time with a larger distance between your dog and your baby. You may want to separate the two by placing your dog in their safe and secure place while rewarding relaxed behaviour. It may help to allow visual contact only with separation, while you work on good things happening when the baby is visible.

 Never leave your baby with your dog unsupervised

Avoid scolding or reprimanding your dog when your baby is present. Your main aim is to foster a good relationship. Make highly enjoyable and fun things happen for your dog whenever your baby is present. If after repeated attempted introductions, even from a distance, your dog will not calm down or consistently shows signs outlined in behaviour group C, then you need to seek assistance from an appropriate veterinarian.

Rarely, some dogs become highly aroused during the introduction and are unable to break from their fixation on the baby. They may become highly focused even to just the sound of the baby, but are often further stimulated by movement too. It is very hard to distract a dog from this focus, and the fixation may occur every time they are in the vicinity of the infant. Dogs displaying these behaviours need to be safely and securely separated from the baby immediately, and advice sought from an appropriate veterinarian.

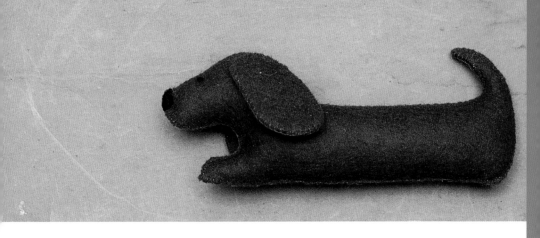

Creating harmony

Your main responsibility is never to leave your baby unsupervised with your dog. Initially, when both partners are home and your dog and baby are together or in the same room, have one partner attend to your baby and the other to your dog. Vary this between the two of you, and try to ensure both partners give your dog equal attention. Try to include your dog in day-to-day activities as much as possible so they do not feel neglected. Do not give your dog attention only when your baby is out of the room and then ignore them when your baby is present. This may cause your dog to associate a lack of attention with the presence of your baby, which is not desirable. Whenever your baby is present, praise your dog and give them tasty food rewards, toys stuffed with food or a chewy treat. Whenever your baby cries, try to remain calm and unrushed to avoid startling your dog.

 If you need to leave the room, separate your baby and dog

When only one of you is home in the first few weeks, and if you do not feel you have good control over your dog, then your dog should be confined to a safe and secure area. It is difficult for one person to monitor everyone in the house all at once. Ideally, this area should enable your dog to see you and your baby, as long as your dog is not showing signs outlined in behaviour groups B or C. Enabling your dog to see the baby and you but still be separated means that you can monitor your dog's response to the baby and also reward them with treats and praise when they are behaving appropriately. Your dog is also likely to remain calmer and feel like a part of the family if they can still see you.

Eventually, your dog may sociably follow you around the house while you attend to your baby. This is fine and helps future interactions between the child and your dog, as long as you can comfortably control your dog with voice commands. If your dog does not respond well to voice commands, they should never be in a situation where they are not safely separated from the baby. If you need to leave the room, safely and securely separate your baby and dog.

Visiting with your baby

Be vigilant of your baby at all times when you visit relatives or friends who own a dog and/or a cat. Their pets may not have had the same exposure to babies and may react differently. It might be helpful to suggest they also use *Tell Your Dog You're Pregnant* or *Tell Your Cat You're Pregnant* before your visit to ensure that their pets are also ready for the new visitor.

Your dog (and baby) sitter

It may be several weeks now since you brought your baby home and you may be thinking about occasionally leaving your baby in the care of a relative, friend or babysitter. It is important not to forget the 'number two' baby now – your dog!

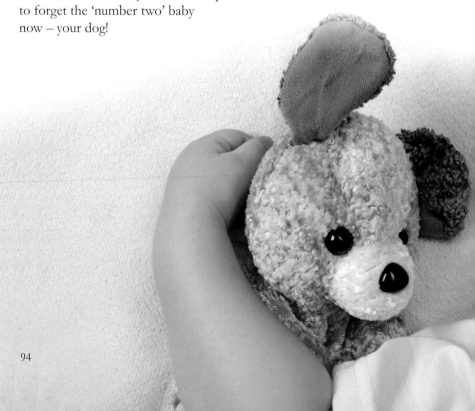

Create a list of checkpoints that pertain to the daily management of your dog. It can be helpful to do this now, even if a babysit is not planned, as it is probable you will be more concerned about your baby's needs and forget to discuss your dog's needs on the actual day. Advanced planning can avoid this.

Things to consider mentioning to the sitter are:

- **Never leave the dog and baby together unsupervised.**
- Use the food rewards provided to reward correct behaviours.
- Ignore any undesirable behaviours or redirect the dog to perform a more desirable behaviour.
- Do not use physical or verbal punishment on the dog.
- Use the same words that you use to instruct the dog (sit, stay, come, drop it, and go to your bed or mat).
- How the dog and baby should be safely and securely separated if the carer needs to leave the room.
- Do not allow the dog in the baby's room when the baby is sleeping.
- Leave the dog alone when they are in their 'safe' dog area.
- Do not disturb the dog when sleeping or eating.
- Do not allow your babysitter to bring unknown dogs into your house when they babysit.

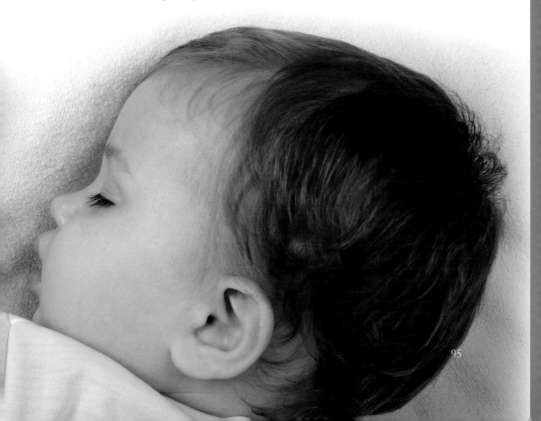

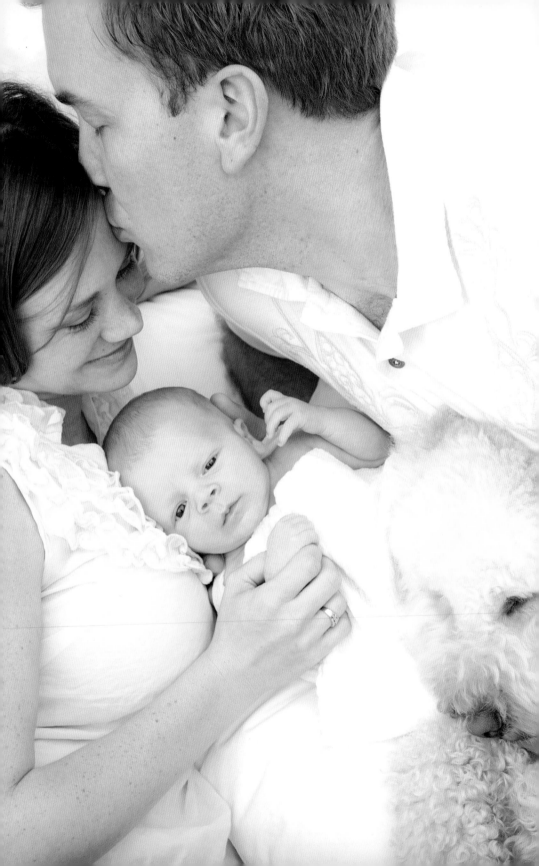

Things to remember

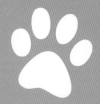

- 🐾 Read the entire book before you start training your dog.
- 🐾 Never leave your baby and dog together unsupervised.
- 🐾 Start preparing your dog as early as possible.
- 🐾 Teach your dog to sit, stay, come, drop it, and go to their bed or mat.
- 🐾 Stop all physical and verbal punishment or reprimands.
- 🐾 Assess how your dog currently reacts around babies.
- 🐾 Create a safe and secure area where you can separate your dog from your baby.
- 🐾 Monitor your dog's body language using behaviour groups A, B and C.
- 🐾 Work slowly through steps 1 to 5 with your dog using the CD tracks.
- 🐾 Distinguish between baby and dog toys to avoid confusion.
- 🐾 Ignore attention-seeking behaviours.
- 🐾 Reward calm and relaxed behaviour.
- 🐾 Set up realistic feeding, walking and play schedules.
- 🐾 Ensure you can control your dog and a pram on walks.
- 🐾 Address any resource guarding and guarding of resting places.
- 🐾 Introduce your dog early to all the new baby-related items in the house and nursery.
- 🐾 Bring home some used baby clothes once your baby is born.
- 🐾 Take the first introduction very slowly. Do not force your dog on your baby or vice versa.
- 🐾 Make fun things happen to your dog whenever the baby is present.
- 🐾 Look forward to the benefits of your extended family.

Further help*

Certain dog behavioural issues are beyond the scope of this book and recommendations have been made to seek professional assistance. Some of these problems are mild and advice can initially be sought from a recommended dog trainer. Other problems are more serious and require assistance from an appropriate veterinarian. An 'appropriate veterinarian' when mentioned in this book is a veterinarian with a professional interest in animal behaviour.

Veterinarians with a professional interest in animal behaviour (appropriate veterinarian)

These are veterinarians that have undertaken further (post-graduate) study or passed examinations in animal behaviour or both. They have a more extensive knowledge than other veterinarians of treating behavioural problems in dogs. They may or may not be veterinary behaviourists.

- Delta Society Australia
  www.deltasociety.com.au/behaviourists
- Australian and New Zealand College of Veterinary Scientists
  www.acvsc.org.au
- American College of Veterinary Behaviorists
  www.dacvb.com
- American Veterinary Society of Animal Behavior
  www.avsabonline.org
- European College of Veterinary Behavioural Medicine
  www.ecawbm.org
- Association of Pet Behaviour Counsellors – United Kingdom
  www.apbc.org.uk

Veterinary behaviourists

These are also veterinarians with a professional interest in animal behaviour but they have undertaken a large amount of further (post-graduate) study in animal behaviour, passed extensive examinations and have met specific criteria, depending on the country, authorising them to use the term 'specialist'.

* Websites listed are for reference only and their content is not endorsed by the author or publisher.

Dog trainers

The dog trainer you consult should be well versed in the latest scientific research on dog behaviour. Years of experience may not always indicate that the trainer uses the most up-to-date methods of training. As discussed earlier, you want to create a harmonious environment for your dog and baby's relationship to develop. For this reason the dog trainer should teach you how to encourage your dog to perform desirable behaviours and then reward them for showing these behaviours. A reward is usually food, pats, verbal praise or play. Unwanted behaviours should be ignored or your dog redirected to perform a different behaviour that is more desirable. Your trainer should use methods that your child, when older, can easily undertake with limited risk of injury. A simple test is to ensure that the methods your dog trainer implements are ones that you would happily use on your own child. Of course you may like to swap the dog treats for lollies!

- Delta Society Australia
  www.dpdta.com.au/trainers
- Association of Pet Dog Trainers Australia
  www.apdt.com.au
- Certification Council for Professional Dog Trainers
  www.ccpdt.org
- Karen Pryor Academy for Animal Training and Behavior
  www.karenpryoracademy.com/find-a-trainer

Behaviour or dog specialists

A quirk of terminology means that anybody who *does not* have a veterinary degree or qualification can actually describe themselves as a 'specialist' or 'expert' regardless of their formal training or experience. Terms often used are:
- dog specialist or behaviourist
- dog behaviour specialist or expert
- animal behaviourist, animal behaviour expert or animal behaviour specialist
- specialist (dog) trainer
- specialising in dog behaviour problems

These people should be judged on their merits as dog trainers, as above.

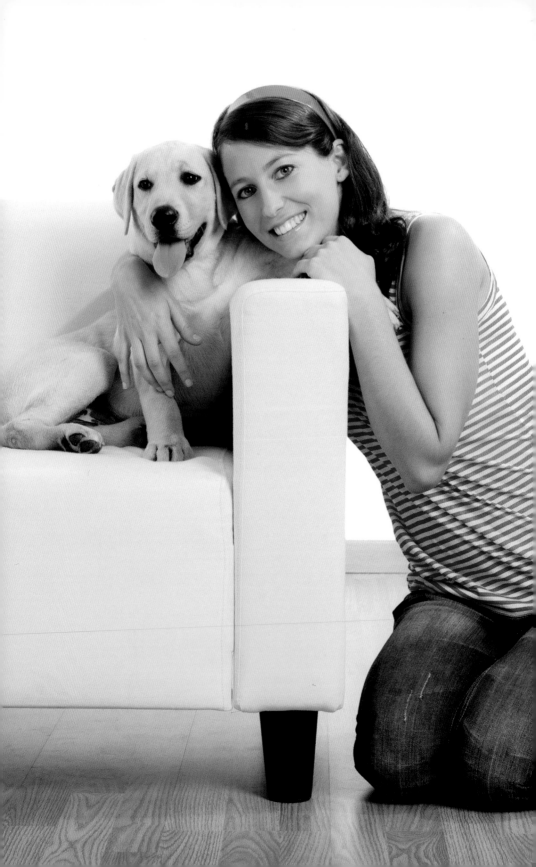

Tell us about your experience

It is hoped that this book has helped you cope easily and smoothly with the addition of another very special member to your family. If you have found this book helpful, please 'like' our Facebook page: **BabyAndPet**. Tell us about your experience or post a photo of your new larger family.

You can also follow the author, Dr Kirkham on Twitter (@VetBehaviourist) for further pet related information.

No photos of unsupervised dogs and babies please!

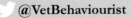 @VetBehaviourist   www.facebook.com/BabyAndPet

www.babyandpet.com.au

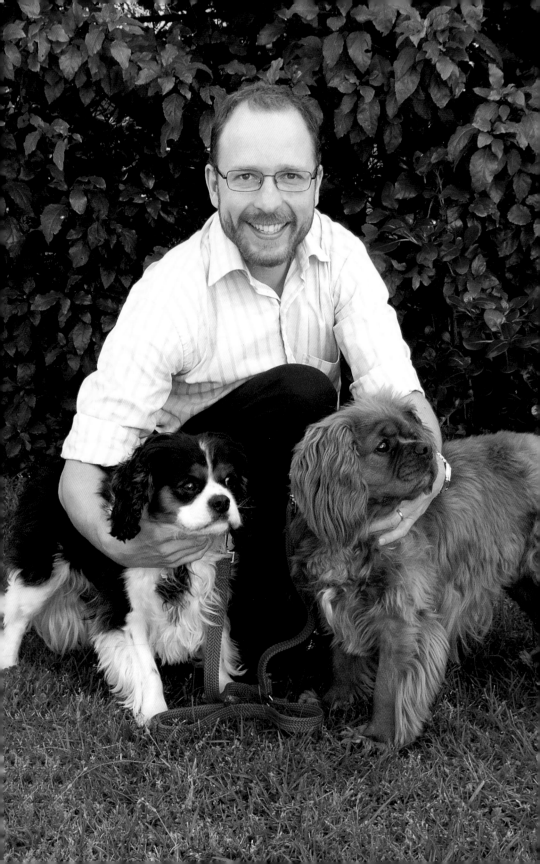

About the author

Dr Lewis Kirkham, a veterinarian with further qualifications in animal behaviour, has a lifelong fascination with pets and their interaction with their owners. Since graduating as a veterinarian from The University of Melbourne in Victoria, Australia, Dr Kirkham has worked in a variety of practices in both Australia and the United Kingdom.

In 2004, he founded Animal Behaviour Solutions, a company that provides private counselling and behavioural advice for pet owners. Through this company, Dr Kirkham has assisted numerous pets and their owners in the assessment and management of behaviour problems. He is also a consultant to local and international zoos and sanctuaries on exotic species' behavioural problems.

Dr Kirkham regularly features on TV, radio and online media regarding behavioural problems in pets. He contributes to *The Age, Herald Sun, The Daily Telegraph, The Courier Mail, The Advertiser* and *The Australian* newspapers, *Dogs Life, Oriental BQ Weekly, Living and Lifestyle* and *Urban Animal* magazines. He has also been published in the *Australian Veterinary Journal*. He is a member of the Australian and New Zealand College of Veterinary Scientists as well as a chartered member of the Australia Veterinary Association. He is also a member of the American Veterinary Society of Animal Behavior.

The birth of his two daughters ignited his passion for educating expectant parents about the smooth transition from a child-free, dog-owning family to a larger family with a new baby. Dr Kirkham's work was initially published as *What your pet can expect when you're expecting* (2005), the first comprehensive resource for expectant families who own a dog or cat. This was re-released in 2012 by Little Creatures Publishing as *Tell Your Dog You're Pregnant: An essential guide for dog owners who are expecting a baby.*

Currently Dr Kirkham divides his time between his family, private veterinary practice, companion and exotic animal behaviour referrals and online veterinary support.

Don't forget your cat!

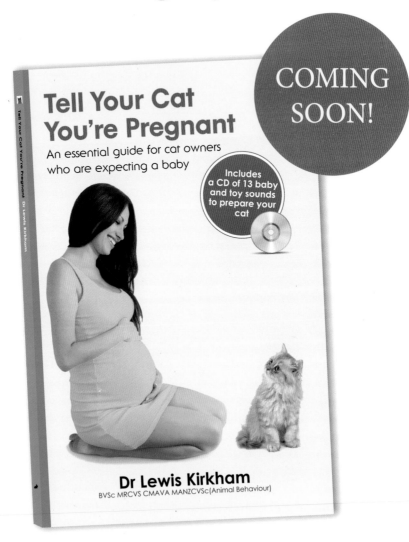

Go to www.babyandpet.com.au for further details